DO NOT REMOVE
CARDS FROM POCKET

ALLEN COUNTY PUBLIC LIBRARY

FORT WAYNE, INDIANA 46802

You may return this book to any agency, branch,
or bookmobile of the Allen County Public Library.

DEMCO

THE PEOPLE'S
SURVIVAL MANUAL

THE PEOPLE'S
SURVIVAL MANUAL

Health Risks
and What
YOU
Can Do About Them

William N. Meshel, M.D.

APPLETON-CENTURY-CROFTS / Norwalk, Connecticut

Copyright © 1982 by APPLETON-CENTURY-CROFTS
A Publishing Division of Prentice-Hall, Inc.

All rights reserved. This book, or any parts thereof,
may not be used or reproduced in any manner without
written permission. For information, address
Appleton-Century-Crofts, 25 Van Zant Street,
East Norwalk, CT 06855

82 83 84 85 86 / 10 9 8 7 6 5 4 3 2 1

Prentice-Hall International, Inc., London
Prentice-Hall of Australia, Pty. Ltd., Sydney
Prentice-Hall of India Private Limited, New Delhi
Prentice-Hall of Japan, Inc., Tokyo
Prentice-Hall of Southeast Asia (Pte.) Ltd., Singapore
Whitehall Books Ltd., Wellington, New Zealand

Library of Congress Cataloging in Publication Data

Meshel, William N., 1946–
  The people's survival manual.

  Includes index.
  1. Cardiovascular system—Diseases—Prevention.
2. Cancer—Prevention.   3. Medicine, Preventive.
4. Health.   I. Title.
RA645.C34M47   616   81-19040
ISBN 0-8385-7822-5   A7822-8 (case)
      0-8385-7821-7   A7821-0 (paper)

Design: Jean M. Sabato

2257799

For my son David

CONTENTS

PREFACE

You have the ability to dramatically change your life expectancy and your susceptibility to the major killer diseases. You are no longer helpless in your own destiny. The knowledge exists that can literally mean the difference between life and death. This book is an attempt to present that information in an understandable, documented, and usable way.

Each year, millions will die of heart disease, strokes, or cancer. Yet scattered throughout the medical literature lies the information that can prevent most of these deaths. Because of the wide range of sources of this information, it is difficult for physicians to be familiar with the many significant factors that can alter their patient's life expectancy. More importantly, there is a great potential health benefit that can result from having this information presented to the American public in an understandable and well-documented fashion.

There have been exciting advances in the diagnosis and treatment of disease in recent years. Despite this, the potential benefit—in terms of the number of lives saved—remains limited. It has recently become recognized that the *prevention* of diseases such as cancer and heart disease would result in the saving of a great many more lives than any therapeutic approach.

Many studies have been undertaken throughout the world to uncover the so-called risk factors that make an individual more susceptible to a particular disease. Protective factors have also been elucidated. If these factors can be modified by large numbers of people, the large-scale prevention of disease becomes a realistic possibility.

Much has been written in the lay press about the prevention of disease. Some of this material is actually misinformation or folk belief.

In other instances the information is accurate, but the perspective is too narrow to accomplish the encompassing goal of prevention. Some authors ask for a mystical or "religious" belief in the wisdom of their thesis. Surprisingly, in other instances, the folk belief presented in these works is actually valid and confirmed by scientific study.

The use of computer searches of the medical literature has made it possible to retrieve data from far-flung studies. Subjecting this data to rigid scrutiny has yielded a solid core of information. This information is presented in this book to allow you, the reader, to take control of your own life. You hold the key to the longevity and health of yourself and your family.

In the first section of the book the United State's major killers, such as heart attack, strokes, and cancer, are discussed. A great deal of information is reviewed in a manner that will allow you to make use of existing knowledge to lessen your risk. The information is extensively footnoted, and references are provided. These references all lead you to articles in highly respected medical and scientific journals. None of these articles is easy for a lay person to read, but you have a right to know the original and rigorous sources for the information presented in this book.

The second section of the book deals with the known major risk factors such as smoking, obesity, stress, alcohol, and coffee. A section that discusses the relationship between drugs, chemicals, food additives, and the development of cancer is also included. The known consequences of these factors are discussed and, some myths about them are dispelled.

The information included in both these sections provides you with a kind of survival manual for today's world. Armed with this information and a concern for yourself and your family, there is much you can do to increase your prospects for good health and a long life.

ACKNOWLEDGMENTS

A great deal of research and effort have gone into the preparation of this book. During those long hours the support—both emotional and technical—of many people was a source of needed sustenance.

Richard Lampert, Editor-in-Chief, Appleton-Century-Crofts, has shown himself to be patient and enlightened. My thanks also to Eileen De Fulgentiis, who never lost hope and laboriously prepared this manuscript. Alice Reilly, the Sippel family, Donna Fenimore, Frank Teller, M.D., Eugene Moran, and Daisy and Murray Levine never waivered in their support.

This text could not have been written without the work of the medical researchers who spend years—often thankless—in the study of the epidemiology of disease.

A special thank you to Miss Linda Cagin, whose love guided me through the dark times and whose patient understanding helped me endure the peculiar loneliness of writing.

INTRODUCTION

As medicine rapidly becomes increasingly sophisticated, it is easy for both physicians and the population as a whole to feel content. After all, what seemed to be science fiction a few years ago is now commonplace. It seemed ridiculous ten years ago to imagine there would be a machine that could take pictures through any "slice" in our bodies without penetration of the skin. Yet such a machine called a CAT scanner (computerized axial tomography) is used routinely, even in some small hospitals. Believing that our technology is a gift that can make us healthier is almost a matter of religious faith. Certainly we can benefit some ill people with our medical skills. Many are saved because of current knowledge. The great epidemics of smallpox, malaria, typhoid, polio, and TB are, thankfully, in most parts of the world a thing of the past. But we are making a deadly mistake!

The same technology that we believe improves our health through better medical care has completely altered our environment, life-styles, diet, and even the very physicochemical structure of the earth's atmosphere. Can any rational person believe these changes are inconsequential?

Each year, millions will die of heart disease, stroke, and cancer. There has been a great deal of well-controlled scientific study supplying much information about these diseases. Although we rapidly utilize this knowledge in the treatment of disease, it is seldom applied to its prevention. We are saving some lives by treatment but losing many more by ignoring prevention.

Surprisingly, perhaps, the government has been in the lead in responding to this "new ball game" in a limited way. The National Institute of Health has funded pilot risk intervention programs. These programs address the issue of preventing disease by modifying some of the predisposing factors associated with them. This is a commendable beginning, but from its conception it perpetuated a major flaw. It is impossible for physicians to "administer" prevention in the same way that antibiotics can be prescribed.

We are at a crossroads in medicine not just because of advances in knowledge but also because of the need for a brand-new philosophy. The time has come for everyone, *you and me,* to become equal partners in assuming responsibility for our health. Mysticism and secrecy in medicine are relics of the past. An educated, aware population is the most important public health measure we can devise.

We are bombarded with confusing, isolated, incoherent bits and pieces of information. It is easy to feel like a helpless victim of circumstance. Television, radio, and newspaper all report that just about everything we eat, drink, touch, smell, and do may cause cancer or heart disease. How can anyone know what to do? Living in a cave in Tibet may seem to be the only way to avoid these dangers.

The current sources of medical information largely fail to supply information adequate to have any real preventive impact. Most of these books deal with poorly documented, sometimes esoteric "solutions" to your problems. These books often have almost cultlike followings. At best, these are often misinformed, and at worst they are written solely with regard to their marketing potential. The other types of books available present relatively sound information but from a narrow perspective. Often they will deal with one of the risk factors associated with disease or at most one particular disease. They are useful but are limited in their perspective and therefore potential benefits.

We live in a time of social change. A newly developed, raised social consciousness is allowing us to reexamine many of the basic, previously unchallenged assumptions of society. We have learned to speak out against war, to break the back of officially sanctioned prejudice, and to question traditional male-female roles and realize the inherent benefit in allowing everyone to realize their potential as productive human beings. Now it is time to realize we can *significantly* improve both the quality and length of our lives. We are not helpless.

This book is an attempt to extract the pertinent, scientifically documented information available in the medical literature and present it in a usable way. It is time to take action and responsibility for your well-being. It can be done! It would be foolishly counterproductive to disregard the real benefits available from existing medical services as well. Both reservoirs of knowledge have merit. The patient and his doctor, working together, can dramatically lower the health dangers an individual faces. Zealots in either camp who deny the value of the other limit the full potential for improving our health.

This book is not a religious work asking for your faith. It is written with personal knowledge of the frustration and futility of failing to resuscitate a heart attack victim or the inability to attain tumor shrinkage in a cancer patient. It is written with a firm belief that there is information available that can literally mean the difference between life and death. It is written with the hope that you will join me and take responsibility for yourself and your well-being. The information provided, utilizing the usual scientific criteria as guidelines, is solidly established. Unsupported theories or techniques are sometimes noted but, when mentioned, are clearly presented as not yet proved. The information provided is documented and footnoted.

The major diseases killing Americans today and the factors that are linked with their development are reviewed. Heart disease, stroke, high blood pressue, pulmonary embolism (blood clot in the lung), breast cancer, lung cancer, and colon cancer are discussed. Separate sections dealing with the effects of smoking, obesity, physical exercise, emotional stress, cancer-causing pollutants and food additives, alcohol and coffee are presented. In this way, information regarding those things that play a causative (or predisposing) role in the major diseases affecting you and me is available. Knowing these so-called risk factors and what steps you can take to decrease your exposure to them can minimize your chances of succumbing to these diseases. Obtaining maximum adequate medical care is an important partner in prevention and health. Therefore, the character and significance of traditional medical care for each disease is touched upon.

You are not helpless in your own destiny. Caring enough about yourself and your family to do something is the sole prerequisite to increase significantly your chance for a longer and healthier life. Use the information provided sensibly and with whatever assistance your physician can provide. Don't accept everything in print automatically. Food fads, gimmicks, and unconventional medicines, including such things as hitherto unidentified vitamins that may be promoted in print, are usually useless and occasionally dangerous. The liquid protein diet that proved to be responsible for several deaths was widely promoted by a doctor's "testimonial" and is an example of the pitfalls faced by an uncritical reader.

Now let's look at what you can do to live longer.

THE PEOPLE'S
SURVIVAL MANUAL

PART ONE

ONE

Heart Attacks

More than 700,000 people will die this year from heart disease, the single largest cause of death in the United States today. It alone accounts for 38 percent of the total deaths reported annually and is responsible for more deaths than the next three leading causes combined: cancer, strokes, and accidents. Deaths from heart attacks are attributable to the heart-muscle damage that results from a relative lack of oxygen to the heart; 44 percent result from heart attacks per se and an equal number from chronic ischemic heart disease, which is heart disease resulting from the long-term deprivation of the heart muscle of its blood supply.[1] The cost in human misery is far greater than such figures reveal when the resulting disability, disruption of family life, and loss of productivity from nonfatal heart disease are added into the equation. It has been noted frequently that heart disease has reached epidemic proportions in the industrialized nations of the world, especially in the United States. Although there is a great deal of sophistication present in the technology that is used to treat patients who enter hospitals with heart attacks, very little has been done from a preventive standpoint. It is now quite clear that it is no longer medically sound to wait until a patient is brought to the emergency room. In such cases, the care given is too little and too late to have any real impact on the problem as it exists today. However, information is available in the medical literature that will enable an individual to protect himself against the ravages of heart disease. It is with this in mind that the present chapter is written.

Coronary artery disease is the underlying cause of heart attacks and chronic ischemic heart disease. The coronary arteries are the blood vessels that supply the nutrients and oxygen to the heart muscle. When there is an imbalance between the ability of these blood vessels to deliver blood supply and the heart muscle's demands, ischemic heart disease may result. If the imbalance is severe enough, there can be actual death of the heart muscle. This occurs in heart attacks that are also termed myocardial infarctions, coronaries, or coronary occlusions. Such terms are all synonymous. When the deficiency of blood supply to the heart muscle is less severe and death of heart tissue does not occur, chest pain, referred to as angina pectoris, may result. Angina pectoris is a very common problem in the United States and is often treated with the drug nitroglycerin, which dilates the blood vessels and allows more blood to reach the heart muscle. (However, it has been suggested that the drug may relieve the pain of angina pectoris through some other as yet undefined mechanism.) Since the root of all these problems is an inadequate blood supply to the heart, it is important to look at the mechanisms by which the heart muscle develops a blood supply insufficient for its metabolic needs.

Vessels that supply the heart muscle are subject to the same degenerative changes that occur in all blood vessels in the rest of the body. These changes can result in narrowing or clogging within the vessel opening. This relative stricture of the vessel can lead to a situation in which less oxygen reaches the heart muscle at any given time. When oxygen delivery to the heart is inadequate for the particular metabolic situation, ischemic heart disease results. If the imbalance between need and supply is great enough, there may be damage and finally death of heart tissue. Medically, the process resulting in such degenerative changes and occlusions of the blood vessels of the body is termed atherosclerosis. Atherosclerosis is a laying down within the vessel walls of fibrous fatty plaques and possibly small blood clots that lead to the occlusion of the blood vessel. The process of atherosclerosis, or hardening of the arteries, is known to be associated with certain disease states, among which are high blood pressure, diabetes mellitus, hypothyroidism (low thyroid), high cholesterol, obesity, and old age.

WHAT ARE THE SYMPTOMS OF HEART DISEASE?

There are many symptoms of heart disease. They result from either inadequate oxygen supply to the heart muscle (myocardial ischemia), inadequate pumping ability of the heart, or abnormal heart rate or rhythm. Myocardial ischemia is most often expressed as chest pain. This pain is characteristically pressure or "viselike" and often radiates into the jaw or arm. Recurrent episodes of this type of pain are what is known as angina pectoris. Persistence of this pain over a period greater than a few minutes may indicate a heart attack. Characteristic of the chest pain associated with heart disease is its association with increased activity or exertion and its lessening or disappearance with rest. This pain can also commonly be experienced after eating. Heart attack pain can also be associated with sweating and nausea. Although there are many other causes of chest pain, some of which are very minor medical problems, it is safest to have a physician investigate any episode of chest pain.

Inadequate pumping by the heart muscle can be manifested by weakness, increased tiredness, dizziness, blood pressure drop, and abnormal retention of fluid (swollen ankles, fluid in lungs, inability to lie flat without becoming short of breath, difficult breathing). Many of these symptoms are seen in other diseases; for example, difficulty in breathing can be seen in obesity, lung disease, and anxiety.

Abnormal rates or rhythms can give rise to the rapid onset of symptoms, which can include fainting, palpitations, difficulty in breathing, and blood pressure drop. Commonly, these symptoms disappear as rapidly as they appear; occasionally, they may persist.

Symptoms are the common warning signs of many different disease processes. They must be interpreted by a physician in light of his clinical expertise and with the help of electrocardiograms (EKGs), chest x-rays, stress testing, and, possibly, other techniques, which will be discussed later.

HOW YOU CAN REDUCE YOUR RISK

The most important step is to prevent the changes that occur in the walls of the blood vessels supplying the heart muscle. There is encouraging evidence, however, from animal experiments that even after such changes have occurred, they may not progress further and may even improve if certain factors are changed. Knowledge of the risk factors not only should enable an individual to increase his "survival" chances but also should allow health professionals to identify those individuals at risk. This, in turn, might produce large-scale risk intervention programs as a very important public health tool. Until that time arises, however, it is important that each individual take the time to be made aware of what he can do to live longer.

Recognizing the tremendous importance of separating out and identifying those factors that are associated with the development of coronary artery disease, several large studies were begun after World War II. The studies were all prospective or forward looking, that is, they followed large numbers of patients for long periods of time. Most notable are the Framingham Study,[2] Chicago Study, Los Angeles Study, Western Collaborative Study, Minnesota Study, and Chicago Utility Co. Study. Utilizing such sources of information, it is possible to be aware, with some degree of assurance, of the known risk factors and the steps an individual can take to avoid exposure to them.

When these large studies were begun, the factors that had a relationship with heart disease were unknown. Therefore, a great many different variables were analyzed and are still being evaluated. It is fair to say that at this time there is enough information available to make meaningful changes possible and thereby reduce the chances of succumbing to heart disease.

There are several factors known or suspected to be associated with the development of heart disease (Tables 1-1 and 1-2).

CHOLESTEROL

It cannot be coincidental that Americans, who have very high levels of cholesterol, also have a very high incidence of heart disease. The powerful association between cholesterol and atherosclerosis has been

TABLE 1-1. RISK FACTORS ASSOCIATED WITH THE DEVELOPMENT OF HEART DISEASE

Age

Sex

Elevated cholesterol

High blood pressure

Cigarette smoking

Elevated levels of certain fats known as 102-density lipoproteins

Diabetes mellitus

TABLE 1-2. POSSIBLE RISK FACTORS ASSOCIATED WITH THE DEVELOPMENT OF HEART DISEASE

Obesity

Elevated triglycerides

Lack of physical activity

Personality type

Menopause

Blood type

clearly demonstrated. Indeed, cholesterol and elevated blood pressure are the most important risk factors associated with the development of heart disease. The danger of heart disease is proportional to the level of cholesterol even in the low ranges still usually considered normal, the danger accelerating above levels of 200 mg percent. In the Framingham Study, the chances of people having heart attacks between the ages of 30 to 49 with a cholesterol level greater than 260 mg was three to five times greater than the rate of heart attacks in people with cholesterol levels below 220 mg percent.

Cholesterol is essential to the digestion of fats. It is both made in the body and ingested by eating cholesterol-rich foods. The average adult in the United States eats approximately 600 mg of cholesterol and 40 gm of fat per day. There is evidence that alterations of serum cholesterol by changing dietary habits can be very significant; animal studies have shown, in fact, that diet manipulation can actually reverse the already-present pathologic changes in blood vessel walls.[5] Blood cholesterol levels can be lowered with diets low in cholesterol, low in saturated fats, and high in polyunsaturated fats.[6] When the above type of diet is combined with a weight loss, the effect on lowering cholesterol is even greater.[7]

The industrialization and affluence of American society has completely rearranged the American diet in the past 100 years. The amount of saturated fats, refined sugar, cholesterol, and salt in our diet have all been dramatically increased, while at the same time opportunities for physical activity and exercise have been sharply reduced.

Animal products are the sole source of cholesterol in our diets. Butter, milk, cream, eggs, meat, and cheese all have large amounts of cholesterol. Egg yolks and organ meats (liver, kidney, and sweetbreads) have the highest cholesterol content of all. Although seafood is generally thought of as safe, in fact, shrimp, lobster, and clams are all high in cholesterol.

What You Can Do About Cholesterol

There are simple steps that can be taken to lower the saturated fat and cholesterol content of your diet:

1. Eat lean meat; trim all the fat from the meat before cooking. When purchasing ground meat, have the meat trimmed and then ground. Attempt to avoid liver, kidneys, sweetbreads, hot dogs, bologna, caviar, luncheon meats, and other combination meats.
2. Fish and poultry should be substituted for beef as often as possible. Poultry skin should be avoided.
3. Veal can be substituted for beef. Although veal does contain cholesterol, it has less saturated fat than beef.
4. Decrease your ingestion of eggs.
5. Butter can be substituted with vegetable oils or margarine high in polyunsaturated fats. Good examples are safflower oil, soy bean oil, corn oil, and cotton seed oil. Palm oil and coconut oil should be avoided.
6. Substitute skim milk for whole milk when possible.
7. Remember, fruits and vegetables have no cholesterol, and they are completely safe to eat.

8. Pocket cholesterol counters are available and are very reasonable. Investing in them is a good way to learn what foods are rich in cholesterol and what foods are not.

9. See your physician and determine your baseline cholesterol and fat levels, including a "lipid profile." (This will be explained later in the chapter.)

10. Adjust your caloric intake to achieve and maintain ideal weight.

The accompanying table (Table 1-3) shows both the saturated fat and cholesterol content of certain selected fats.[8]

Drugs that have sometimes been used to lower serum cholesterol are clofibrate (Atromid-S) and nicotinic acid. The benefit of these drugs in preventing heart disease has not been well established. Their use should be determined by your physician in light of his knowledge of your blood chemistries and overall physical status.

HIGH BLOOD PRESSURE

The most powerful risk factor in the development of heart attacks is high blood pressure.[9] Elevated blood pressure in a person with high cholesterol is particularly devastating. Both of these risk factors have been shown to interact in a way that reinforces their potential damage to blood vessel walls. Experiments have clearly demonstrated that high blood pressure in animals on high cholesterol diets produces much more narrowing of the blood vessels supplying the heart than high cholesterol diets in animals with normal blood pressure.[10] Unlike other risk factors evaluated, the damaging effect of high blood pressure was seen in both sexes and in all age groups.[4]

High blood pressure, or hypertension, is a common problem affecting more than 20 million Americans. Blood pressure is simply the force with which the blood courses through the vessels of the body. There is no difference between blood pressure and the water pressure that develops in any pipe system. In the former case, the pipes are represented by the blood vessels of the body. The pressure head that occurs is the result of the power with which the heart pumps the blood and the relative elasticity of the blood vessel walls. The more rigid the blood vessel walls, the greater the force that is necessary for the blood to flow through them and reach the tissues that they supply. The con-

TABLE 1-3. DIETARY FAT REGULATION—FATTY ACID AND CHOLESTEROL CONTENT OF SELECTED FOODS*

| Foods | Portion | | Total Fat, gm | Fatty Acids | | | Choles-terol, mg |
	Amount	Weight gm		Saturated, gm	Monoun-saturated (oleic), gm	Polyun-saturated (linoleic), gm	
Milk, Cheese, Eggs							
Buttermilk, cultured, from skim milk	1 cup	246	trace	…	…	…	0.7
Dry, nonfat	1 cup	80	1	…	…	…	8.4
Fluid, nonfat	1 cup	246	trace	…	…	…	0.7
Cottage cheese, from skim milk							
creamed	1 cup	225	11	6	4	trace	79
uncreamed	1 cup	225	1	trace	trace	trace	1.1
Eggs, large, 24 oz per doz.							
Raw whole, without shell	1 egg	50	6	2	3	trace	340
white of egg	1 white	33	trace	…	…	…	…
Meat, Poultry, Fish, Shellfish							
Beef, trimmed to retail basis, cooked. Cuts braised, simmered, or pot roasted, lean only	2.5 oz	72	5	2	2	trace	90
Roast, oven cooked, no liquid added, lean only (round)	2.5 oz	72	4	2	2	trace	45

Food	Amount						
Chicken, cooked, canned, boneless	2.8 oz	79	12	3	6	2	72
	3 oz	85	7	2	3	1	76
Lamb, trimmed to retail basis, cooked leg, roasted, lean only	2.5 oz	72	5	3	2	trace	56
Pork, cured, cooked ham, smoked, lean, and fat	3 oz	85	24	9	10	2	107
Pork, fresh, trimmed to retail basis, cooked: roast, oven cooked, no liquid added, lean only	2.4 oz	68	10	4	4	1	66
Cuts simmered, lean only	2.2 oz	63	6	2	3	1	62
Veal, cooked, cutlets, broiled, without bone	3 oz	85	9	4	4	trace	72
Bluefish, baked or broiled	3 oz	85	4	(...)	(...)	(...)	(...)
Clams, raw, meat only	3 oz	85	1	(...)	(...)	(...)	103
Crabmeat, canned or cooked	3 oz	85	2	(...)	(...)	(...)	(...)
Haddock, fried	3 oz	85	5	1	3	trace	54
Mackerel, broiled, Atlantic	3 oz	85	13	(...)	(...)	(...)	63
Ocean perch, breaded (egg and breadcrumbs) fried	3 oz	85	11	(...)	(...)	(...)	(...)
Oysters, meat only, raw 13–19 medium selects	1 cup	240	4	(...)	(...)	(...)	280

(continued)

TABLE 1-3 (continued)

| Foods | Portion | | Total Fat, gm | Fatty Acids | | | Choles-terol, mg |
	Amount	Weight gm		Saturated, gm	Monoun-saturated (oleic), gm	Polyun-saturated (linoleic), gm	
Salmon, pink, canned	3 oz	85	5	1	1	(...)	55
Sardines, Atlantic type, canned in oil, drained solids	3 oz	85	9	2	2	4	59
Shad, baked	3 oz	85	10	(...)	(...)	(...)	(...)
Shrimp, canned, meat only	3 oz	85	1	(...)	(...)	(...)	118
Tuna, canned in oil, drained solids	3 oz	85	7	2	1	4	43
Nuts							
Almonds, shelled	1 cup	142	77	6	52	15	...
Brazil nuts, broken pieces	1 cup	140	92	18	44	24	...
Peanut butter	1 tbsp	16	8	2	4	2	...
Pecans, halves	1 cup	108	77	5	49	15	...
Walnuts, shelled, black or native, chopped	1 cup	126	75	4	26	36	...
Vegetable Products							
Potato chips, medium, 2-in diameter, fried in vegetable oil	10 chips	20	7	2	2	4	...

Grain Products

Food	Measure						
Cracked-wheat bread	1 slice	23	.5	...	...	...	(...)
Italian bread, enriched	1 slice	23	.2	...	...	...	...
White bread, enriched, 1 to 2%, nonfat dry milk	1 slice	23	1	...	...	...	...
Whole-wheat, graham, entire-wheat bread	1 slice	23	.7	...	...	...	...
Cakes:							
Angel food, sector, 2 in. (1/12 of 8-in diameter cake)	1 sector	40	trace	...	...	...	...
Sponge cake, sector, 2 in. (1/12 of 8 in. diameter cake)	1 sector	40	2	1	1	trace	110
Cornmeal, white or yellow, dry, whole, ground	1 cup	118	5	1	2	2	...
Macaroni, enriched, cooked	1 cup	130	1	...	...	2	(...)
Noodles (egg noodles) enriched, cooked	1 cup	160	2	1	1	trace	(...)
Oatmeal or rolled oats, regular or quick cooking, cooked	1 cup	236	3	1	1	1	(...)
Rice, white, cooked	1 cup	168	trace	...	...	...	...
Spaghetti, enriched, cooked	1 cup	140	1	...	...	...	(...)
Wheat flours, whole wheat, from hard wheats	1 cup	120	2	trace	1	1	...

(continued)

13

TABLE 1-3 (continued)

Foods	Portion Amount	Weight gm	Total Fat, gm	Saturated, gm	Monoun-saturated (oleic), gm	Polyun-saturated (linoleic), gm	Choles-terol, mg
All-purpose or family flour, enriched, sifted	1 cup	110	1	...	...	...	...
Fats, Oils							
Special margarine (range)	1 tbsp	15	12	(14–28)	(18–42)	(22–34)	...
Oils, salad or cooking							
corn	1 tbsp	14	14	2	4	7	...
cottonseed	1 tbsp	14	14	3	3	7	...
olive	1 tbsp	14	14	2	11	1	...
safflower	1 tbsp	14	14	1.7	1.8	10.5	...
soybean	1 tbsp	14	14	2	3	8	...
Salad dressings, commercial, plain mayonnaise type,							
4 percent egg	1 tbsp	15	6	1	1	3	4
French	1 tbsp	15	6	1	1	3	...
mayonnaise, commercial	1 tbsp	15	12	2	3	6	4

...: not present.
(...): data not available.
*Data from Kritchevsky D, Tepper SA, Hayes OB, Rose G

cept of rigidity of blood vessels is reflected by the term *peripheral resistance.* In high blood pressure, peripheral resistance is increased. There are other factors besides the nature of the blood vessel walls that play a part in the development of hypertension. It has recently been shown that both blood volume and sodium retention play important roles in blood pressure elevations. High blood pressure has been shown to shorten the life span of patients. The higher the pressure, the more the life span is decreased. Before the development of effective treatment for high blood pressure, the average life of an untreated individual was 20 years from the date of diagnosis. Some of the most common causes of death in these untreated people were: heart failure, stroke, heart attack, and kidney failure.

The great majority of people with high blood pressure have no symptoms. Headaches, although popularly thought of as common with hypertension, are typical only in persons with very highly elevated pressures. Typically, the headache is described as occurring in the back of the head and is present upon awakening in the morning. Identification of people with high blood pressure usually occurs during a routine physical examination.

The therapy used to lower blood pressure has been shown to be effective in lowering the incidence of many of the complications of the elevated pressure.[11] It has not yet been demonstrated to lower the risk of heart attack. Despite this, a preponderance of evidence and logic speaks of the importance of lowering blood pressure. Its status as an important risk factor is clear.

What You Can Do About High Blood Pressure

1. Getting regular checkups by your physician is the only way to allow for early diagnosis and treatment. Early treatment is important because it is in the early stages of high blood pressure, before damage to the heart, brain, and kidney occurs, that significant prophylaxis can occur.

2. The relief of emotional and environmental stress is considered an important measure in lowering blood pressure. Patients admitted to hospitals with high blood pressure are frequently noted to have lower pressures 3 or 4 days after admission without any treatment. This is presumed to be from the alleviation of their usual environmental stress.

3. Diet and salt restriction are useful in lowering blood pressure. In obese patients, they can be combined with caloric restriction. As previously mentioned, diets low in cholesterol and saturated fat are important.
4. Regular exercise has been shown to help weight control and actually lower blood pressure.
5. Weight reduction in a controlled study was demonstrated to effect highly significant improvement in blood pressure control.[12]
6. Very effective drug therapy is available for lowering blood pressure with a minimum of side effects. First-line therapy usually involves a diuretic, a drug that induces the body to eliminate excess fluids.

The important thing to remember is that elevated blood pressure is a killer and usually has no obvious symptoms. If your doctor puts you on a medication, take it even though you may feel fine. One of the difficulties many doctors experience in treating patients with high blood pressure is the tendency in patients to stop taking medication when they feel well. This can be a very serious mistake and can have important implications for the future well-being of that patient.

There are many possible side effects associated with taking medications to control your blood pressure. Symptoms such as lightheadedness, weakness, nausea, insomnia, and depression are associated with the various drugs used to control high blood pressure. If you have any side effects, it is important to see your physician, but remember: *Don't stop taking your medicine.*

CIGARETTE SMOKING

Smoking is strongly implicated as a risk factor in many different diseases. Men who smoke one pack of cigarettes per day have a 70 percent greater chance of dying from heart disease and have twice as great a likelihood of developing heart disease.[13] There is also a greater incidence of heart disease in women smokers, although the associated risk is not as great as that seen in men. Pipe and cigar smoking seem to have less importance, although they also' increase the risk of heart disease. The incidence of sudden death has also been shown to be strongly associated with smoking, and the greater the amount of cigarette smoking, the greater the death rate. It is encouraging, however, that in people who stop smoking, sudden deaths and heart attacks are approximately one-half those who continue.[4] There has been some confusion and controversy regarding what the mechanism is through which smoking exerts its effect on the incidence of heart disease. There have been several interesting theories proposed to explain the increase in heart disease that accompanies smoking.

It is known that the nicotine in cigarettes can cause elevations in blood pressure and a more rapid heart rate. This increase in blood pressure and heart rate causes the heart to work harder. The result of the increased heart work means that the heart muscle needs a greater oxygen supply. Worsening the situation, smoking cigarettes, regardless of their nicotine content, causes elevations of the substance known as carboxyhemoglobin. Carboxyhemoglobin is formed when the hemoglobin in the blood, which usually binds oxygen and is used to carry oxygen in the blood to the tissues, preferentially binds up carbon monoxide. This happens because hemoglobin actually has a much greater affinity for carbon monoxide.

However, since carboxyhemoglobin is not capable of transporting needed oxygen, a relative decrease in oxygen supply to the heart results. Therefore, a situation develops in which the heart needs more oxygen and in fact is able to receive less than usual. The literature discusses specific mechanisms in an attempt to explain the increase in heart attacks and sudden death in cigarette smokers. They include the following:[14]

1. Nicotine increases the heart muscle's need for oxygen, probably through the already-mentioned mechanism of increasing cardiac work and rate.
2. Nicotine increases the tendency to form blood clots. Blood clots may be implicated in the occlusion of the vessels supplying blood to the heart.
3. Nicotine lowers the threshold for developing dangerous heart rhythms. The development of dangerous rhythms is probably the mechanism through which sudden death occurs. Certain cardiac abnormal rhythms can lead to death because of the heart's inability to function and pump blood efficiently.
4. Carboxyhemoglobin interferes with the delivery of oxygen to the heart.

5. Carboxyhemoglobin lowers the heart muscle's strength of contractions.
6. Carboxyhemoglobin also lowers the threshold for dangerous heart rhythms.
7. Carboxyhemoglobin also increases the blood's tendency to clot.

It has been reported that carboxyhemoglobin is found in increased amounts in nonsmokers who are simply sitting next to smokers. This concept is known as "passive smoking," and its effects would indicate that there is indeed importance to the current movement to restrict smoking.

Smokers have more hardening of the arteries than nonsmokers, and when the heart's blood vessels and muscle were examined, there were greater changes in smokers than in nonsmokers. The changes were also greater in people who smoke many cigarettes, than in those who smoke a lesser number. Specifically, at the level of the smallest arteries in the heart, which are known as arterioles, there was advanced degeneration found. It was noted in 90.7 percent of those smoking two or more packs a day, in 48.4 percent of those smoking less than one pack a day, and not in one person who was a nonsmoker.[15]

It is clear that smoking increases the risk of heart attack and heart disease. Unfortunately, it is also clear that being around smokers may also increase that risk.

What You Can Do About Cigarette Smoking

1. Stop smoking. There are many programs, both public and private, that attempt to help smokers do this. They use different techniques, such as hypnosis, and have varying rates of success. In the United States today there are many programs and booklets which try to help stop smoking and educate school children before they begin.
2. If you can't stop smoking, decrease the amount. There is clear evidence to show that the less you smoke, the better off you are.
3. Switch from cigarette smoking to a pipe or cigar, which are safer with respect to heart attacks and heart disease.

However, it should be remembered that they are not at all safe with regard to lip and mouth cancers.

ELEVATED FATS AND LOW-DENSITY LIPOPROTEINS

The importance of serum cholesterol as a risk factor is well established. Cholesterol and fats can be partitioned into various lipoprotein patterns. Lipoproteins are the forms in which all fats, except for free fatty acids, are present in the blood plasma. Fat and cholesterol are linked to proteins for transport. Fats are known as lipids and since they are combined with proteins, the term lipoprotein simply refers to the combined vehicle of fat, cholesterol, and proteins that are used to transport these substances in the blood. Cholesterol is partitioned among these various factions.

Briefly, here is what happens to fat in the body: Fats leave the stomach and are mixed with bile and an enzyme produced by the pancreas known as "pancreatic lipase." Bile is secreted by the gall bladder and acts on the large fat particles to make them soluble. These bile salts make the lipids available to be absorbed. All the fats enter, circulate, and leave the blood bound to specific proteins. Lipoproteins are the principal transporters of lipids in the blood. Lipoproteins can be spun down and separated into components that differ on the basis of their density. When these are separated, they are broken down into high-density lipoprotein (HDL), low-density lipoprotein (LDL), very low density lipoprotein (VLDL), and chylomicrons. VLDL is made in the liver and is broken down into LDL and HDL. When the risk of heart disease is considered, looking at the fractions of lipoproteins involved, some interesting information is learned: LDL appears to be very dangerous, while HDL exerts a protective effect. VLDL has no apparent separate effect. All this, at first, might seem confusing; it simply means that cholesterol in the form of LDL has a deleterious effect, while in the form of HDL, for some reason, there is a protective effect. This protective effect in HDL may explain why some patients with a high total cholesterol do much better than others with a similarly high cholesterol. In other words, if the total cholesterol has a significant proportion in HDL, it is not as important a risk as it would be if it were all in LDL. However, levels of LDL do correlate with levels of total cholesterol. What this means is that the higher your total cholersterol is, probably the higher your LDL is.

In evaluation of 2815 men and women aged 49 to 82, HDL had the largest impact on the risk of heart disease.[16] This impact was protective, that is, the higher the HDL levels, the less the risk. Whereas persons with low HDL levels had greater risks, persons with HDL levels less than 35 mg had eight times the risk of persons with HDL levels of 65 mg or higher.

Information concerning your body's fractionation of lipids can be obtained when your doctor orders a blood test called a "lipid profile." It is evident that this fractionation of total cholesterol into HDL and LDL and VLDL is very important and can give a more clear understanding of what your risks are of developing heart disease. This will allow your doctor to predict more correctly what the chances are of your succumbing to heart disease.

What You Can Do About HDL Levels

Measures you can take to lower your total cholesterol have already been discussed. Now let's look at what can be done to change the proportions of HDL (the protective factor). HDL levels are known to correlate inversely with weight, triglycerides, and diabetes and to correlate directly with physical activity. In other words, if you are overweight, have a high triglyceride level or diabetes, you probably have a lower HDL. On the other hand, if you exercise, your HDL levels are higher. Although it has not been documented, it would seem likely that you can raise your HDL levels and therefore reduce your risk by:

1. Losing weight
2. Exercise, being careful not to overdo it
3. Eating low cholesterol, low saturated fat diets to decrease your LDL

PHYSICAL ACTIVITY

The relationship between physical activity and heart disease has long been suspected. Evidence now available clearly implicates lack of physical activity as a risk factor. In a large prospective study, death from heart attacks, cardiovascular deaths, and, indeed, the overall death rate were related to physical activity.[2]

It is also apparent that people in good physical condition have a better chance of surviving a heart attack if they develop one. Studies have also been done comparing other risk factors in people with varying physical conditions. These studies show that serum cholesterol, blood pressure, triglycerides, and percentage body fat were all related to physical activity.[17] All these factors improved with improving physical condition. Physical conditioning is now clearly established as a way to reduce the chances of your dying from heart disease. It is important to remember to exercise in a program that is suited to your physical condition. Excessive strenuous exercise can be dangerous.

MENOPAUSE

It is well known that women have a decided advantage over men with regard to the risk of developing heart disease. This biologic protective mechanism seems to lose its effect with advancing age, so that the incidence of heart attacks in older women approaches that seen in men. Since this protective effect occurs during the reproductive years, the association of heart disease with menopause has been evaluated in a large study.[2,18] Within the same age group, 40 to 54, women who underwent menopause had a three times greater chance of developing cardiovascular disease. The advantage of premenopausal women disappears with menopause and in women whose husbands developed heart disease. In women whose husbands developed heart disease, the incidence of heart attacks was much greater regardless of menopausal status. This latter finding demonstrates clearly the important influence of environmental factors.

BLOOD TYPE

Curiously, blood type appears to have a relationship to the development of certain cardiovascular diseases. People with blood type O seem to have a lower risk. This was significant statistically with regard to the medical problem known as "intermittent claudication," seen commonly as leg cramps due to decreased blood flow to the body's muscles. There is no clear explanation as to why blood type O would have some protective effect in this disease. Although in other cardiovascular diseases the results were not statistically significant, there is also a trend toward lesser risk of other diseases such as stroke and heart attack with blood type O. It has been postulated that this might result from some effect of this blood type on clotting.

PERSONALITY TYPE

Personality type has been popularly espoused as a risk factor in the development of heart disease. This has not been clearly shown. In this schema, the "high-strung, uptight" individual allegedly has a greater chance of having a heart attack. No definite statement regarding this as a risk factor per se can be made. However, this personality type probably is associated with other risk factors such as smoking and sedentary life-style.

ALCOHOL

There is no apparent increased risk with regard to cardiovascular diseases and alcohol consumption. Reports in the literature have suggested both an increased risk and a lowered risk in drinkers. The preponderance of evidence, however, supports no relationship, and in heavy drinkers there is actually the suggestion of protective benefit.[19] This should by no means be construed as suggesting that excessive alcohol intake is beneficial. Clearly, the overall effect of alcohol on disease and physical condition is a deleterious one. Alcohol is associated with many other diseases, including liver damage and damage to the nervous system.

COFFEE

Coffee has long been suspected as a risk factor in heart disease. Recent evidence has shown that this is not the case. There is no apparent relationship between coffee intake and any of the cardiovascular diseases.

NEW FRONTIERS

The search for the isolation and detection of risk factors continues. Preventive drug therapy with various agents such as thyroid hormones, estrogen, aspirin, sulfinpyrazone (Anturane), and others has also been an area of interest.

Aspirin has been extensively evaluated in the coronary drug project research group.[20] This study evaluated more than 1500 men who had previous heart attacks. The group treated with aspirin had 30 percent less deaths, which is very suggestive of a beneficial effect of aspirin on heart attacks but is not statistically conclusive. There is some evidence suggesting that aspirin may play a preventative role in the development of another cardiovascular disease, stroke, in males. Additionally, it is very important to remember that the chronic use of a medication like aspirin may be dangerous. Aspirin, although it is popularly considered safe, can have very serious effects, including bleeding and ulcers. More information is needed to conclude that aspirin is beneficial in heart attacks.

A very exciting new development is taking place with the drug sulfinpyrazone (Anturane); sulfinpyrazone has been used since 1959 for the treatment of gout. It, like aspirin, interferes with the ability of the blood to clot. Since the formation of small blood clots in the blood vessels of the heart may play a role in heart attacks and in sudden death, it has been the object of a multicenter clinical trial.[21]

Patients with recent heart attacks were entered into this study. The results were so striking that the trial sponsors reported them early. There was a decrease of 48.5 percent in heart-related deaths with the drug-treated group. When the rate of sudden deaths were compared, the sulfinpyrazone group had a 57.2 percent decrease compared to controls. This may have significant implications in the prevention of death from heart attacks. Currently, this study is being continued for a more complete evaluation.

YOU AND YOUR DOCTOR

Although this chapter discusses many factors that can be altered to decrease the risk of having a heart attack, there is still an important need for medical attention. Your physician can provide you with the advice and valuable information you need to know to best protect yourself. Some of the procedures that give useful diagnostic information are discussed below; these procedures, when used together with a complete history and physical, allow for a highly accurate assessment of the clinical situation and your risks.

Chest X-rays

Chest x-rays can give information about the condition of your heart, lungs, and the blood vessels in the chest. They provide an accurate assessment of heart size and the presence or absence of enlargement of the chambers of the heart. Heart failure, as well as degenerative changes in the large blood vessels, can be readily noted. Chest x-rays are also important in that they are permanent records that can be used for future comparisons.

Electrocardiograms

The electrocardiogram (EKG) is a graphic recording of the electrical activity of the heart taken during each beat. These electrical patterns or waves can be correlated with known disease states and abnormal situations. The EKG is obtained by applying metal electrodes to the skin in specific anatomic locations. These electrodes are then attached by wires to a recording machine. The recording can then give information about the heart rate and rhythm: electrical activity, chamber size, conductivity of the heart and heart muscle, lack of oxygen, damage from a new or previous heart attack, certain drug effects, salt imbalances, to mention just a few. In many cases of heart attacks, the EKG changes are obvious. However, a heart attack can occur with no changes in the EKG or changes that may not evolve for days. Helpful in assessing the damage done from heart attacks are changes in cardiac enzymes. (See below.)

Enzymes

In situations in which damage has been done to the heart muscle, there is an associated rise of certain enzymes. The enzymes commonly used to monitor heart damage are: CPK, SGOT, and LDH. Changes in these enzymes must be interpreted in the light of the clinical situation since they may also become elevated in other situations.

Stress Test

This is a very useful test and is a good office screening procedure as part of a routine physical for persons at risk. An EKG is taken while a person is exercising. The stress of exercise may elicit EKG abnormalities that are not seen on the resting EKG.

Special Studies

Further diagnostic tests are available if the routine studies are not adequate.

Cardiac catheterization. A procedure in which a small tube can be passed through a vein or an artery to the right or left side of the heart, respectively. The small tube allows pressure measurements in the various chambers of the heart. It can be used to calculate the functional integrity of the various heart valves, the presence or absence of certain abnormalities in the heart, and other abnormalities of heart function. A dye can be injected through this tube into the various chambers of the heart, and the tube can be threaded into the coronary arteries, which are the blood vessels supplying oxygen to the heart muscle. This will allow a graphic representation of the patency of the vessels supplying the heart muscle. Cardiac catheterization can provide information that is useful in many situations and is routinely done prior to any open heart procedures.

Echocardiogram. A painless technique that bounces sound waves off the structures of the heart and great vessels. The theory behind the technique is not different from that of radar or sonar. It allows visualization of the movement of the various heart structures and can be interpreted to give valuable information about the heart structure and function. Much of the information gained with this technique could previously have only been gotten with cardiac catheterization.

WHAT DOES THIS ALL MEAN?

Heart disease is a vicious killer and crippler, but it is one that can be stopped. The information contained in this chapter can be used intelligently and with the advice of your doctor can decrease substantially the chances of your having a heart attack or becoming a victim of heart disease. It is important at this point to reiterate that self-medication with any of the drugs discussed, exercise that is not reasonable for your physical conditioning, and fad diets can be very dangerous. Certainly, the recent deaths from the liquid protein diets should be striking enough evidence that a sensible diet and exercise program must be worked out with your physician with knowledge of your physical condition and biochemical parameters. Smoking or changing your diet may not be easy, but living as a crippled victim of heart disease or leaving behind a widowed family is the alternative. The time to do something about heart disease is *now*. Waiting until symptoms develop is too late.

REFERENCES

1. Vital Statistics Report; *DHEW Publication No.* (PHS) 78–1120, vol. 25, no. 13, December 1977, pp. 1–29.
2. Kannel William B: Recent findings from the Framingham Study—1. *Medical Times* April 1978, pp. 23–27.
3. Glueck Charles J., Mattson Fred, Bierman Edwin L: Diet and coronary heart disease: another view. *New England Journal of Medicine* 298:1471–1474.
4. Kannel William B: "Further Findings from Framingham." *Medical Times* May 1978, pp. 97–103.
5. Armstrong ML, Warner ED, Connor W E: Regression of coronary atheromatrics in rhesus monkeys. *Circulation Research* 2759, 1970.
6. Rifkind BM, Levy, RL (eds): *Hyperlipidemia: Diagnosis and Therapy.* New York, Grune and Stratton, 1977.
7. Ashley FW, Kannel WB: Relation of weight change to changes in atherogenic traits: the Framingham Study. *Journal of Chronic Diseases* 27:103–114, 1974.
8. White P: The regulation of dietary fat. *JAMA* 181:411–429.
9. Kannel WB: The role of cholesterol in coronary atherogenesis. *Medical Clinics of North America* 58: 363–379, 1974.
10. Hollander William, Madoff I, Paddock J, et al. Aggravation of atherosclerosis by hypertension in a subhuman primate model with coarctation of the aorta. *Circulation Research* 38 (June suppl) 11-63–11-72, 1976.
11. Freis Edward D: Effects of treatment on morbidity in hypertension. *JAMA* 213: 116–122, 1143–1152, 1970.
12. Ramsey LE, Ramsay MH, Hettiarachihi J, et al: Weight reduction in a blood pressure clinic. *British Medical Journal* 2:244–245, 1978.
13. Wintrobe MM, et al (eds): *Principles of Internal Medicine.* New York, McGraw Hill, p. 1306.
14. Aronow Wilbert S: Effect of cigarette smoking and of carbon monoxide on coronary heart disease. *Chest* 70: 514–518, 1976.
15. Auerbach Oscar, Carter Harry W, Garfinkel MA, et al: Cigarette smoking and coronary artery disease. *Chest* 70: 697–705, 1976.
16. Gordon Tavia, Costelli William P, Hjortland Marthana C, et al: High density lipoprotein as a protective factor against coronary heart disease. *American Journal of Medicine* 62: 707–714, 1977.

17. Copper Kenneth H, Pollock Michael L, Martin Randolph P, et al: Physical fitness levels vs. selected coronary risk factors *JAMA* 236: 166–169, 1976.

18. Kannel William B, Hjortland Marthana C, McNamara Patricia M, et al: *Annals of Internal Medicine* 85: 447–452, 1976.

19. Stason William B, Neff Raymond K, Miettinen Ollie S, et al: Alcohol, consumption and nonfatal myocardial infarction. *American Journal of Epidemiology* 104: 603–608, 1976.

20. Wilkens Robert W, et al: Aspirin in coronary heart disease. *Journal of Chronic Diseases* 29: 625–642, 1976.

21. Sherry S, et al: Sulfinpyrazone in the prevention of cardiac death after myocardial infarction. *New England Journal of Medicine* 298: 289–295, 1978.

TWO

Strokes

Stroke is the third largest cause of death in the United States and takes a heavy toll upon Americans. Only heart disease and cancer cause more death and disability. As more and more people live to older ages, stroke has become a major public health issue with important economic, social, and medical consequences. There will be 500,000 new strokes this year, causing 200,000 deaths. It is estimated that 1.6 million Americans suffer with varying degrees of disability from stroke, with 640,000 requiring special care and 160,000 of these needing total supportive care.[1]

WHAT CAUSES A STROKE?

A stroke is typified by the rapid onset and development of symptoms that result from brain damage. The specific symptoms depend on the size, shape, and location of the damage. Damage and disability from a stroke can range from very slight to severe, with accompanying paralysis and coma. The severe form has also been called apoplexy, shock or cerebrovascular accident. Strokes can cause paralysis, numbness, loss of sensation, inability to talk, blindness, blurred vision, dizziness, difficulty swallowing, coma, and many other abnormalities.

Stroke occurs when the brain tissue is deprived of its oxygen supply. Oxygen is transported in the blood and travels through two main arteries on each side of the neck, known as the carotid arteries and vertebral arteries, to reach the brain. Any disease process or physical condition that decreases the flow of blood to the brain can cause a stroke. The amount of damage that occurs depends on the severity, location, and duration of the inadequate blood flow.

There are several different mechanisms that can cause interference with the blood supply to the brain. Atherosclerotic thrombosis is hardening of the arteries that can affect the vessels supplying the brain. Blood clots form at the site where blood vessels are narrowed. This can lead to a blockage of the vessel and a reduction of the amount of blood reaching the brain. The brain tissue supplied by that vessel becomes "starved" and eventually dies. The varied symptoms that can result depend on which blood vessel is blocked and which areas of the brain are therefore damaged.

Another important way in which stroke can occur is known as cerebral embolism. A blood clot, either from the heart or from an artery, breaks loose and is swept with the blood toward the brain. It continues traveling in the blood vessels of the brain until it lodges in a vessel with an opening too small for it to pass. This clot may then obstruct the flow of blood to that area of the brain.

The third most common pathway in the development of stroke is intracranial hemorrhage, or bleeding in the head. There are two main types of bleeding that may occur. The first is bleeding into the substance of the brain as a result of high blood pressure. This is termed hypertensive intracerebral hemorrhage. The other type of bleeding results from the rupture of a weakened wall of a blood vessel in the brain. This weakened wall is referred to as an aneurysm.

After the onset of a stroke, the victim's condition can either stabilize, worsen, and eventually lead to coma and death, or improve partially or totally. The degree of brain damage that can follow a stroke is highly variable. If the decrease in blood supply is temporary and minimal, a "transient ischemic attack" (TIA) occurs. TIAs used to be known as "little strokes." These little strokes have symptoms similar to stroke, but they disappear within 24 hours. Their importance is that they may be a warning sign of impending stroke. On the other end of the spectrum, deprivation of the brain's blood flow can lead to the phenomenon of sudden death. Sudden death is any death that occurs less than 24 hours after the onset of symptoms and for which there is no known preexisting illness or event. Stroke accounts for 10 to 20 percent of all sudden deaths. In investigating this problem, a review of the records of the residents of Rochester, Minnesota, from 1955 to 1969, revealed that bleeding into the brain was responsible for all but two cases of stroke-related sudden death and that 88 percent of these victims had high blood pressure.[2]

Stroke is not only a problem that old people encounter. Sometimes, even children and young adults can have strokes. When young people are afflicted, the cause and outcome differ dramatically from their older counterparts. The association of children and strokes was recently reviewed. The factors causing stroke in this age group are entirely unique. Abnormalities that lead to stroke in children include:[3]

1. Abnormalities of the blood vessels, which can result in sudden paralysis in children. This is named "acute hemiplegia of childhood."
2. Defective blood vessels, allowing bleeding to occur into the brain. These defects are termed "arteriovenous malformations."
3. Congenital heart disease. This is heart disease that results from an inherited abnormality.
4. Obstruction of the venous drainage from the head by an infected blood clot. This is known as "purulent venous thrombosis" and can follow infection of the mastoid, sinuses, or scalp.
5. Injury to the head.
6. Sickle cell anemia.

Young adults between the ages of 8 and 40 who developed stroke were evaluated in a similar fashion. In 55 percent of these patients, the underlying cause could be identified. Many of these patients had blood clots that arose from the heart lodged in the brain's arteries. In the under-30 age group, the preponderance of stroke was in females. It is postulated that this prevalence of females in the under-30 group may be the result of their utilizing birth control pills, which are known to increase the risk of blood clots. In the group of young adults aged 8 to 40, high blood pressure was the most significant influencing factor. Overall, younger patients did better in recuperating, with 75 percent improving and becoming independent.[4]

The problem of stroke is a serious one. Since brain tissue cannot repair itself, the damage that results from a completely evolved stroke is permanent. Once present, this damage is, as expected, not very responsive to any medical manipulations. Therefore, it is important to shift our emphasis to the prevention of stroke. Stroke, after all, is the result of many years of exposure to many risk factors. The most promising approach available to lessen the impact of this disease involves determining the risk factors and intervening.

WHAT ARE THE RISK FACTORS FOR STROKE?

There have been many large studies attempting to determine the risk factors in stroke. Since hardening of the arteries is a common mechanism in both heart attacks and stroke, it was thought that the risk factors for both diseases would be similar. Studies designed to obtain etiologic factors in strokes followed designs similar to the large heart disease studies.

In the Framingham Study, 5184 men and women aged 30 to 62 were followed for 22 years.[5] Of this group, 294 developed stroke. Hardening of the arteries with the formation of blood clots was the most common cause of stroke with 59 percent of the cases, blood clots to the brain were responsible for 14 percent, and bleeding into the head caused 15 percent. Analysis of the data revealed important information. Unlike heart disease, men and women were equally at risk. (The protective effect for heart disease seen in premenopausal women was not operative in stroke.) The important risk factors identified were age, high blood pressure, level of blood hemoglobin, heart disease, and diabetes mellitus. Cigarette smoking, obesity, physical activity, level of cholesterol, tea, coffee, dietary habits, and alcohol were unimportant factors in the development of stroke.

High blood pressure is the single most potent and significant precursor leading to stroke. The higher the blood pressure either systolic or diastolic (first and second number), the greater the risk of stroke. This holds true in both men and women in all age groups. Only 15 percent of people with stroke had normal blood pressures.[1] Many studies have confirmed the association of high blood pressure with stroke.[5-9]

It has been argued that treating high blood pressure may actually result in lowering the amount of blood flow to the brain because of an inadequate pressure. This postulated decrease in cerebral blood flow could therefore exacerbate the deficiency of oxygen to the brain, resulting in a worse situation. However, recent evidence shows there is actually an increase in blood flow to the brain and clinical improvement with treatment for high blood pressure.[10] Patients with high blood pressure under treatment have fewer strokes. A postmortem evaluation of patients who had low blood pressure episodes confirms that low blood pressure is not a significant factor in precipitating strokes in patients with hardening of the arteries that supply the brain.[11]

Heart disease is strongly associated with the risk of having a stroke. Previous heart attack victims, people with a history of heart failure, or people with certain abnormalities that show up on their EKG have a higher risk. People who have had a heart attack are three times more likely to have stroke than other people.[1]

Cigarette smoking, although an important risk factor in heart disease, and peripheral vascular disease (lack of oxygen supply to the extremities resulting in pain) have no clear relationship to stroke. There is no difference in the risk of developing stroke in smokers and nonsmokers.

A high cholesterol level has a very minimal effect as a risk factor for stroke. Although it is an important precursor to the hardening of the arteries that supply the heart as seen in heart disease, it does not have the same influence on the development of strokes.

Diabetes mellitus is associated with an increased risk of stroke in both men and women.

Hemoglobin is the component of blood that chemically links with oxygen and acts as a chemical vehicle to transport it to the cells of the body. The risk of stroke is greater when the hemoglobin level is above 15 mg/100 ml in men and 14 mg/100 ml in women.[12] This risk was confirmed in a study of 432 patients who had post-mortem examinations.[11] Smoking and high blood pressure can increase hemoglobin levels.

WHAT YOU CAN DO ABOUT STROKE

Factors that can be modified are high blood pressure, heart disease, and diabetes mellitus. Diabetes mellitus can often be improved simply by weight reduction with caloric restriction.

High blood pressure can be easily treated with a low salt diet and appropriate drugs. The usual first-line drug in the treatment of high blood pressure is a once-daily diuretic (water pill). The chances of developing heart disease can be definitely lessened. The risk factors that are known afford an individual the opportunity to decrease markedly his risk. (See Chap. 1.)

The changes in your life-style that will minimize the risk of becoming a stroke victim should be started as early as possible. The changes in the blood vessels supplying the heart and brain begin early in life.

The development of symptoms of TIAs is in fact an early warning system that can alert you and your physician to the high risk you face of developing a stroke. Knowledge of the significance of TIAs has led some medical investigators to attempt to intervene in the progression of the disease at this point.

In an attempt to assess the possibility of surgical intervention to remove a blood clot from the artery it blocks, 123 patients were studied. Dye was injected into blood vessels to determine how large and where the occlusion was; 89 percent of these patients had demonstrable blockage, with 71 percent in a location amenable to surgery. The investigators feel surgical intervention can stop TIA episodes and prevent stroke.[13]

Others have suggested treating TIAs with blood thinners (anticoagulants). The idea here is to inhibit the formation of blood clots and thereby avoid blockage of an artery. In one study, 199 patients with TIAs were treated with blood thinners. The results from the study show no difference in survival between the treated and untreated group. However, the recurrence of TIAs was significantly less after 3 months of treatment. Unfortunately, this study notes an increase in the incidence of bleeding into the brain in people treated with blood thinners.[14] Another study used blood thinners to treat 178 people with TIAs. The investigators concluded that patients treated with blood thinners seemed to be protected against strokes. They recommend lifelong anticoagulation for patients with a blockage in the carotid artery and at least 1 year of treatment when the basilar artery is obstructed.[15]

Acting on information provided by Health, Education and Welfare in 775 TIA victims that the probability of stroke following TIA was estimated at 20 percent in the first year and 45 percent within 5 years, another study was begun. The investigation, in an attempt to improve the statistics, took 45 patients with TIAs and aggressively intervened in every possible risk factor over a 5-year period.

Patients with elevated cholesterols and fats were placed on diets that restricted animal fats and eggs. Diabetics were placed on the American Diabetic Association diet. Patients with operable blockage had surgery. Patients with heart disease were treated with drugs. Patients with increased hemoglobin were bled to lower their hemoglobin. Emotional stress was treated with counseling and sedation. Cigarette smoking was stopped by many participants. Obese patients were put on caloric restricted diets. Patients with high blood pressure were treated. Finally, patients with high uric acid levels were put on drugs and special diets. Although there is no evidence that all these variables are risk factors, such intervention decreased the incidence of stroke to 7 percent compared to a projected 45 percent.[16]

The value of surgery in these patients is not clearly determined. Reports in medical journals differ with regard to the success rate and the incidence of death and disability related to surgery. Surgery has been used in TIAs, bruits (noisy blood flow over the carotid artery, indicating turbulence secondary to obstruction), and recent stroke. The literature notes that success rates in cleaning out the blood vessels range from 20 to 64 percent. Death related to surgery was highest in patients with recent strokes.

In one study of 40 patients, who were divided into low and high surgical risks, there were no deaths in the low-risk group.[17] Patients were considered high-risk if one of the following were applicable:

Neurologic. Large amount of brain functional damage that is less than 2 weeks old, progressively evolving stroke and minimal brain damage less than 24 hours.

Medical. History of heart attack, heart failure, obesity, old age, high blood pressure.

The investigator concludes that using these criteria, low-risk patients should be operated on.

Another surgical study with 228 patients showed a 41.7 percent death rate from surgery in patients with severe stroke and a 21.1 percent death rate in patients operated on with TIAs.[18] This high death rate gives some perspectives on the dangers that are inherent in this surgery.

DRUG THERAPY

Many drugs have been studied in an effort to influence either the occurrence or evolution of stroke:

Nicotinic acid is a drug that dilates the blood vessels. It was tested in an attempt to increase blood flow to the brain but was shown to have no effect on cerebral blood flow. Hydergine, Dexamethasone, and Mannitol are all drugs that reputedly reduced the swelling that accompanies stroke. In a controlled study, none of the drugs had any beneficial effect.[19]

Sulfinpyrazone interferes with the ability of the blood to clot. This property of sulfinpyrazone led to its being tried in 585 patients in an attempt to alter the risk of recurrent stroke or death. It was not found to be effective.[20]

NEW FRONTIERS

Ironically, one of the most exciting new developments in attempts to reduce the death and recurrent stroke rates in people with TIAs involves the very old and common drug aspirin. Aspirin interferes with the ability of the blood to clot. A study of 178 patients treated with aspirin for 37 months showed equivocal benefit.[21] A second study with 586 patients yielded dramatic results. Male patients with threatened stroke had a 48 percent decrease in the death and recurrent stroke rates.[19] Aspirin has a significant impact on survival and disability for males with TIAs. Unfortunately, this protective effect is not seen in women.

YOU AND YOUR DOCTOR

Regular visits to your doctor are an integral part of a comprehensive program to decrease your risk. High blood pressure, a significant risk factor in stroke, is usually asymptomatic and needs to be checked regularly. Reducing your risk of heart disease is also an important factor in avoiding strokes. In order to do this, your doctor can provide you with information you need, including lipid profiles, EKG, recommended diet, and appropriate exercise. Some useful medical tests that may be obtained to evaluate strokes are briefly discussed below.

Lumbar Puncture
A needle is placed in the back to sample the fluid surrounding the brain and spinal cord. Information about the nature of the stroke can be obtained from the opening pressure, blood count, chemistries, and color of the fluid.

Skull X-rays
A picture of the integrity of the bony skull is provided that can also be used to determine a shift in the position of the intracranial contents.

Angiography
A flexible tube is passed into either a large artery of the neck or one in the elbow or groin. The site can then be injected with dye to visualize the arch of the aorta, the major blood vessels feeding the brain (the carotid or basilar arteries), and eventually the very small arteries that branch off from the larger ones. This can demonstrate blocked vessels, tumors, bleeding into the brain, and pockets of infection.

Radioactive Isotopes (Brain Scan)
Radioactive isotopes of mercury, technetium, or arsenic can be used to visualize tumors, pockets of infection, large blood clots, and sometimes abnormal blood vessel structures. It is a simple and painless procedure.

CAT Scan
The CAT scan is a new radiologic technique. Information from 30,000 beams of x-rays is interpreted via computer and gives pictures of "slices" through the brain. This has been shown superior to brain scans in detecting blood clots in the brain substance.[22]

Electroencephalograph (EEG)
Electrodes are placed in the scalp and the EEG machine records graphically the electrical activity of the brain. Certain manipulations are carried out that may give additional information about the way the

brain is functioning. The manipulations include deep breathing, flashing lights, and sleep. EEGs can give information on epilepsy, brain tumors, large blood clots, pockets of infection, drug usage, and space-occupying masses.

The key to avoiding the potentially devastating effects of stroke is to act now.

1. See your doctor regularly.
2. If you have high blood pressure, take your medication.
3. Avoid the risk factors associated with heart disease.
4. If you tend to be diabetic, lose weight.
5. Check your blood hemoglobin (routine part of a blood count).

Waiting until there are symptoms or brain damage from a stroke is too late. Remember brain tissue does not regenerate.

REFERENCES

1. Wolf Philip A, Dawber Thomas R, Thomas Emerson H, et al: Epidemiology of stroke. *Advances in Neurology* 16: 5–19, 1977.
2. Phillips II Lawrence H, Whisnant Jack P, Reagan Thomas J: Sudden death from stroke. *Stroke*, 8: 392–395, 1977.
3. Golden Gerald S: Strokes in childhood and adolescents. *Stroke,* 9: 169–171, 1978.
4. Grindal Alan B, Cohen Robert J, Saul Robert E, et al: Cerebral infarction in young adults. *Stroke* 9: 39–42, 1978.
5. Kuller Lewis H: Epidemiology of cardiovascular diseases: current perspectives. *American Journal of Epidemiology* 104: 425–456.
6. Librach Gershon, Schadel Meir, Seltzer Moshe, et al: Stroke: incidence and risk factors. *Geriatrics* 85–96, 1977.
7. Stolley PO, Kuller LH, Nefzger MD, et al: Three-area epidemiology study of geographic differences in stroke mortality. *Stroke* 8: 551–557, 1977.
8. Rabkin Simon W, Mathewson Francis AL, Tate Robert B: Long term changes in blood pressure and risk of cerebrovascular disease. *Stroke* 9: 319–327, 1978.
9. Okada Hiroshi, Horibe Hiroshi, Ohno Yoshiyuki, et al: A prospective study of cerebrovascular disease in Japanese rural communities, Akabane and Asaki. *Stroke* 7: 599–607, 1976.
10. Kannel William B, Dawber Thomas R, Sorlie Paul, et al: Components of

blood pressure and risk of atherothrombotic brain infarction: the Framingham Study. 7: 327–331, 1976.

11. Torvik A, Skullerud K: How often are brain infarcts caused by hypotensive episodes? *Stroke* 7: 255–257, 1976.

12. Tohgi Hideo, Yamanouchi Horoshi, Murakami Mototaka, et al: Importance of the hematocrit as a risk factor in cerebral infarction. *Stroke* 9: 369–374, 1978.

13. Eisenberg Ronald L, Nemzek William R, Moore Wesley S, et al: Relationship of transient ischemic attacks and angiographically demonstrable lesions of carotid artery. *Stroke* 8: 483–486, 1977.

14. Whisnant Jack P, Cartlidge Niall EF, Elveback Lila R: Carotid and vertebral-basilar transient ischemic attacks: effect of anticoagulants, hypertension, and cardiac disorders on survival and stroke occurrence — a population study. *Annals of Neurology* 3: 107–115, 1978.

15. Olsson Jan E, Muller Ragnor, Berneli Sune: Long term anticoagulant therapy for TIAs and minor strokes with minimum residuum. *Stroke* 7:444–451, 1976.

16. Leonberg Stanley C, Elliott Frank A: Preventing Stroke after TIA: *American Family* 17: 179–183, 1978.

17. Kusunaki T, Rowed DW, Tator CH, et al: Thromboendarterectomy for total occulsion of the internal carotid artery: a reappraisal of risks, success rate and potential benefits. *Stroke* 9: 34–38, 1978.

18. Easton Donald J, Sherman David G: Stroke and mortality rate in carotid endarterectomy: 228 consecutive operations. *Stroke* 8:565–568, 1977.

19. Santambrogio Sergio, Martinotti Renato, Sardella Francesco, et al: Is there a real treatment for stroke? Clinical and statistical comparison of different treatments in 300 patients. *Stroke* 9: 130–132, 1978.

20. Barnett HJM, A randomized trial of aspirin and sulfinpyrazone in threatened stroke: *New England Journal of Medicine* 299: 53–59, 1978.

21. Fields William S, Lemak Noreen A, Frankowski Ralph F, et al: Controlled trial of aspirin in cerebral ischemia. *Stroke* 8: 301–314, 1977.

22. Gado Mokhtar, Coleman Edward R, Merlis Anthony L, et al: Comparison of computerized tomography and radionuclide imaging in "stroke." *Stroke* 7: 109–113, 1976.

THREE

High Blood Pressure

High blood pressure can kill you. It is very widespread in Western societies and quite deadly. Happily, there is a great deal you can do to protect yourself and your family. It is now believed that in most cases high blood pressure can be prevented entirely. Furthermore, if you already have high blood pressure, you can help yourself a great deal.

More than 15 percent of the adult population of the United States — some 23 million people — have high blood pressure, making it the most common cardiovascular disorder seen by practicing physicians.[1] Only one-third or less of the high blood pressure victims have adequate control of their high blood pressure, and 5 million are not even aware they have the problem.[2] Insurance companies have long been aware that high blood pressure shortens the life span. Indeed, the higher the blood pressure, the shorter your life expectancy. Before the advent of effective drug therapy, the life expectancy of the average untreated patient was 20 years. These people succumbed to the damage that organs and blood vessels received at the hands of the increased pressure. The most common causes of death were heart failure, strokes, heart attacks, kidney failure, and rupture of the aorta (the major artery in the body).

Worsening the problem and contrary to popular belief, the majority of people with high blood pressure have no warning signs or symptoms. Headaches, although commonly believed to be prevalent with high blood pressure, are characteristic only with severe high pressure. High blood pressure is a proven risk factor in heart disease and strokes (two of the leading three causes of death in the United States). In a study of 5209 men and women followed for 20 years, people in the age range of 35 to 64 with high blood pressure had three times the occurrence of heart disease, four times the risk of developing heart failure, and seven times the risk of stroke.[3]

High blood pressure is a serious and common problem. Treatment is important, but prevention has largely been ignored. There are now enough accumulated data to allow a realistic attempt to prevent high blood pressure. Some investigators believe that the incidence of high blood pressure can be dramatically reduced and even eliminated as a major public health problem.[4]

WHAT IS HIGH BLOOD PRESSURE?

Blood pressure is the force with which the blood courses through the vessels of the body. High blood pressure, or hypertension, is a relatively consistent elevation in this pressure above normal levels. The pressure head that develops within the blood vessels is not all that different from the water pressure in a plumbing system. In the case of blood pressure, the pipes are the blood vessels, and the pump is the heart. The pressure generated is a result of the force with which the heart pumps and the elasticity of the blood vessel walls. When the blood vessel resistance to blood flow is abnormally high, the blood pressure rises. A specific cause for this elevation in resistance cannot be found in approximately 90 percent of patients with high blood pressure. This is termed essential or idiopathic hypertension. When a cause for the elevated blood pressure can be found, it is known as secondary hypertension.

Blood pressure readings have two parts, systolic and diastolic. The first number (systolic pressure) is the blood pressure obtained during contraction of the heart. The second number (diastolic pressure) is the blood pressure obtained during relaxation of the heart. The blood pressure is recorded as two numbers; for example, in 130/80, the first number is the systolic pressure and the second is the diastolic pressure. These numbers are recorded in millimeters of mercury, a pressure unit used frequently in scientific work.

The goal of treatment is to lower the blood pressure to more nearly normal levels. This is done in an attempt to avoid the harmful effects that can result from an elevated blood pressure. There are many studies that clearly show that even mild high blood pressure bodes unfavorably in terms of total death rate, death from heart disease, and stroke.[5] One leading investigator reviewing his extensive data considered high blood pressure the most common and potent risk factor contributing to cardiovascular death.[6] Whether treatment of high blood pressure decreased this risk used to be the subject of some medical debate. It has been shown now in several studies that lowering blood pressure really does reduce this risk. Two studies carried out by Veterans Administration physicians showed benefits in treating both mild and moderate high blood pressure.[7,8] In another study, treatment of high blood pressure was recently shown to lower both the total death rate and the rate of fatal and nonfatal heart attacks in middle-aged men.[9]

It is now well established that high blood pressure is deleterious to your health and that lowering this pressure is beneficial. Fortunately, in most cases, the pressure can be lowered readily. The particular diet and/or drug regimen most appropriate for you must be individualized. Again, your doctor is a key partner in helping you prevent the increased risk you face if you have high blood pressure. Sometimes it is hard to understand the importance of taking medications when you feel fine. Remember the damage that can occur with high blood pressure often occurs without aches or pains.

After clinical evaluation and laboratory tests, your doctor may determine there is an underlying disease causing your high blood pressure. As was mentioned earlier, this is true in one case out of ten. Some of the causes of this type of blood pressure elevation include:

1. Diseases of the kidneys or their blood supply
2. Narrowing of the aorta (the major artery in the body)
3. A tumor of the adrenal gland called pheochromocytoma

4. Overactivity or tumor of the adrenal gland producing Cushing's syndrome
5. Overactivity or tumor of the adrenal gland producing aldosteronism
6. Toxemia of pregnancy
7. Ingestion of birth control pills
8. Treatment with medications known as steriods
9. Excessive ingestion of licorice.

Whether or not there is an underlying cause can only be determined by your doctor. In some cases, the cause can be treated. In others, it is more reasonable not to attempt to correct the underlying cause. This determination has to weigh carefully the risk of treatment against the potential benefits.

Most people with high blood pressure have no symptoms. The disease is often first discovered during a routine physical examination. In a smaller number of people, there may be symptoms. These can be the result of the damage caused by the elevated blood pressure or manifestations of the underlying disease (in the case of secondary high blood pressure). Symptoms that result from an elevated blood pressure can include: dizziness, palpitations, tiring easily, nosebleeds, blood in the urine, blurred vision, headaches, difficulty breathing, and headaches. When the symptoms are manifestations of an underlying disease, they may include: increased urination, increased thirst and drinking, muscle weakness, weight gain or weight loss, rapid changes in emotion, headaches, palpitations, sweating, and dizziness upon standing up. All these symptoms can be warning signs of many different diseases. Again, your doctor must play a key role in fitting the pieces together.

Let's take a look at some of the things your doctor considers when he makes a decision on your treatment. First there is the concept, already mentioned above, of "risk versus benefit." This is simply another way of your doctor asking himself, "Am I doing more harm than good by treating this patient?" This is an underlying principle of all medical therapeutic decisions. In the equation, the side effects and possible dangers of therapy must be weighed against the potential good of therapy. The Joint National Committee on Detection, Evaluation and Treatment of High Blood Pressure has reported general guidelines on this very issue.[10] (See Table 3-1.)

TABLE 3-1. TREATMENT RECOMMENDATIONS

Average Diastolic (Bottom number) Blood Pressure	Recommended Action
120 or higher	Immediate evaluation and treatment needed
105–119	Treatment needed
90–104	Individualize treatment
under 90	Remeasure blood pressure at yearly intervals

Adapted from the Joint National Committee on Detection, Evaluation and Treatment of High Blood Pressure.

Once your doctor has decided to treat you, remember the following important points about your illness:

1. High blood pressure is a lifelong and potentially deadly disease. There are very real dangers in not treating the problem.
2. Take your medicines as directed every day. This is the only way to maintain control of the elevated pressure.
3. High blood pressure often has no symptoms. You may feel fine, but you must continue taking your medications.
4. Keep regular follow-up appointments with your doctor.

WHAT ARE THE RISK FACTORS FOR HIGH BLOOD PRESSURE?

There is much information in the medical literature concerning the factors that may predispose someone to the development of high blood pressure. There is still a fair amount of debate about the relative importance of some of these risk factors. Some prominent investigators feel modification of these factors can drastically reduce your chances of becoming hypertensive. Contributing elements that are established as risk factors are summarized in Table 3-2.

Sodium intake and its role in the development of high blood pressure as well as its importance in treatment have been the subject of

TABLE 3-2. RISK FACTORS FOR DEVELOPING HIGH BLOOD PRESSURE

Alcohol consumption

Anxiety or stress

Overweight

Salt consumption

Inheritance

Race

Less education

Birth control pills

debate since the turn of the century. In a recent review of the many existing studies, one investigator has drawn the compelling conclusion that dietary sodium intake is a very significant factor in the development of high blood pressure.[11] He also notes that our dietary sodium intake is a habit acquired from infancy. Reasoning further, he suggests that if families with a history of high blood pressure would reduce their sodium intake, high blood pressure may become much less common. Numerous data support this point of view. In one study of patients with essential high blood pressure, patients could be divided into "salt sensitive" and "nonsalt sensitive" groups.[12] The "salt sensitive" patients responded to an increase in dietary salt with an increase in blood pressure. Also, it is well known that dietary sodium restriction as well as water pills (diuretics), which cause loss of salt through urination, lower blood pressure.

Many studies indicate that anxiety, stress, or anger are factors predisposing to the development of high blood pressure.[13] Some study results have yielded differing conclusions. One recent study concludes that both anger and anxiety can elevate blood pressure in some people, with anxiety being the more significant factor.[14] Somewhat contradictory results have been recently shown in a study in which patients with high blood pressure were noted to have less psychological distress than other patients.[15] However, the available evidence lends itself to the conclusion that daily psychological stress from such factors as urban crowding, military combat, natural catastrophes, noise, and work conditions is an important factor in the development of high blood pressure in some people. Inheritance plays an important role in your chances of becoming hypertensive. In a fashion not unlike the way a tendency toward a certain range of height is transferred from parents to child, you receive a disposition toward certain blood pressure levels at birth. The full impact of this disposition is not yet defined quantitatively. Investigators have stated that from 30 to 80 percent of blood pressure variability is inherited.[16] The authors of a recent review article on the heritability of blood pressure sum up the situation very aptly: "Clearly the best precaution a newborn baby can take over its arterial blood pressure and therefore, its cardiovascular risk in later life is to choose its parents carefully."[17]

Alcohol has been shown in several studies to have an association with high blood pressure.[18–20] In these studies, hypertension was seen almost twice as often in those people who drank more than the average. One large study related blood pressure to known drinking habits in 83,947 men and women.[21] These authors concluded that there is a "strong possibility that regular use of alcohol in amounts above an unknown threshold results in higher blood pressure in a large proportion of patients." In this study, people who said they drank three or more drinks per day were noted to have higher blood pressures.

Obesity has also been noted to have an association with high blood pressure. More obese people have high blood pressure than do nonobese, and more hypertensives are obese. In one study in which 5127 men and women were followed, this association was well demonstrated.[22] The authors of that paper stated, "Adiposity predisposes and makes a significant contribution to development of hypertension in adult men and women beyond age 30." In an excellent review of the extensive data that interrelates high blood pressure and being overweight, the authors made the following points:[23]

1. The association between body weight and high blood pressure is real.
2. Weight reduction has been shown to lower blood pressure.
3. Control of obesity should be an intrinsic part of any therapeutic or preventive antihypertensive regimen.

Thus, the medical literature clearly demonstrates that your being overweight can lead to the development of high blood pressure. It is also reported that overweight hypertensive people have a greater risk of heart disease or stroke than persons with either high blood pressure or obesity alone.

Radical differences in the prevalence of high blood pressure are striking. There are many studies that show that a considerably higher proportion of blacks than whites in the United States have hypertension.[24-26] One study utilizing data from 14 U.S. communities and involving 158,906 adults found 18.0 percent of whites and 37.4 percent of blacks to have high blood pressure. The reasons for these observed differences are not clear. However, there are many contributing variables including diet, weight, and social psychological stress. These and perhaps some as yet undefined influences probably account for racial differences in the prevalence of hypertension.

Level of education, apparently, as a socioeconomic marker also has a relationship to the prevalence of high blood pressure. Data from one of the largest community-based screening and hypertensive treatment programs in the United States revealed that education was inversely associated with high blood pressures. The explanation for this is not obvious but probably has to do with the differences in life-style, diet, stress, and weight that may occur with different levels of educational achievement. Education, in this way, is actually an indication of socioeconomic status.

Birth control pills have added a new dimension to the consideration of risk factors in women. These pills are known to be capable of minimally elevating blood pressure, which alone may not be significant. However, they also can affect blood lipid and blood sugar levels.

The entire situation has been recently reviewed in an editorial by one of the masters of the risk factor medical literature.[27] This review makes several interesting observations:

1. Females have relative immunity from heart and blood vessel disease compared to men at the same age.
2. There are a few things that can eliminate this advantage, including: sugar diabetes, inheritance of abnormal blood-fat levels, advanced age, and menopause.
3. Birth control pills may present a new and as yet unknown risk to women.

4. Birth control pills have an adverse effect on blood pressure, blood fats, and blood sugar.
5. Although the relative risk in users is large, the absolute risk for women under 40 is small. This risk may be lower than the risk of unwanted pregnancy.
6. The final outcome is still unknown. It is not yet clear what changes in risk result from a few decades of exposure.

Thus, it seems that the potential risk to women taking birth control pills is still not clearly defined.

Some of the factors that are commonly believed to exacerbate the risk toward the development of high blood pressure have not been shown to play a causative role (Table 3-3). Smoking and coffee, although indicated as risk factors in other diseases, are not associated with the development of high blood pressure.[28, 29]

TABLE 3-3. FACTORS NOT ASSOCIATED WITH RISK OF DEVELOPING HIGH BLOOD PRESSURE

Coffee

Smoking

WHAT YOU CAN DO ABOUT HIGH BLOOD PRESSURE

From the material already presented, two things become clear. In the first place high blood pressure is dangerous and is a major factor contributing to death and illness in the United States. Second, some of the risk factors already discussed can be altered by changes in your life-style. (See Table 3-4.)

Sodium restriction (especially in the form of table salt) is apparently valuable in both preventing and treating high blood pressure. In one study of hypertensive patients, the blood-pressure-lowering effect of salt restriction was very similar to that obtained utilizing one drug.[30] Table 3-5 lists some of the foods to avoid in a low sodium diet. Although it is not easy in our society to avoid salt since it is almost omnipresent, you can still accomplish a reduction in salt intake by exercising a little care and avoiding the addition of salt to your foods.

TABLE 3-4. WHAT YOU CAN DO TO LESSEN YOUR RISK OF DEVELOPING HIGH BLOOD PRESSURE

Lose weight

Eat a low sodium diet

Exercise

Practice relaxation techniques

Try biofeedback

TABLE 3-5. FOODS TO AVOID IN LOW SALT DIETS

Category	Avoid
Meat	Meat, fish, or poultry that is smoked, brine cured, salted, dried, or canned, including frankfurters, canned beef, chipped dried beef, luncheon meats, ham, salt pork, sausage, salted codfish, sardines
Breads and cereals	Breads, rolls, or crackers with salted tops, pretzels
Butter or other fats	Bacon, bacon fat, roquefort and Thousand Islands salad dressing
Other foods	Bouillon cubes, prepared soup bases, olives, pickles, relishes, salted popcorn, potato chips, sauerkraut
Seasonings	Salts: regular, celery, onion, garlic
Meat flavorings	Some of the available flavorings and tenderizers
Miscellaneous	Prepared mustard, horseradish, catsup, chili sauce, monosodium glutamate (MSG)

Adapted from "Diet Manual for Small Hospitals and Nursing Homes." Publication of Nutrition Section, Wisconsin Division of Health, Box 309, Madison, Wisconsin 53701.

Some investigators feel this alone could dramatically reduce your chances of becoming hypertensive.

Weight reduction is an essential part of any therapeutic or preventive antihypertensive regimen.[31] Not only can weight reduction lower your blood pressure, it can also lower the risk of your developing heart disease if you have high blood pressure. Obese people with high blood pressure have more heart disease than obese people alone or hypertensives alone. Reasonable caloric restriction with the advice of your doctor is the appropriate and safe way to lose weight. Avoid fad diets or crash diets; they can be dangerous.

Exercise has been shown to lower blood pressure in some middle-aged men with high blood pressure. In one study, patients walked or jogged 30 to 35 minutes twice a week. In six months, their blood pressure was lowered an average of 13 to 12 mm Hg.[32] A similar result was obtained in a Canadian study. Thus, exercise is a helpful way to reduce the risk you face from high blood pressure. Any exercise program should be undertaken with the advice of your doctor — don't overdo it.

Relaxation techniques, including transcendental meditation, have been shown capable of lowering blood pressure in hypertensive patients. The long-term benefit of such techniques has not yet been established. However, they appear to be useful in coping with the stress of society.

Biofeedback has also been shown capable of temporarily lowering blood pressure. Its long-term usefulness is not established.

Drug Therapy

The purpose of drug therapy in the treatment of hypertension is to use a drug, alone or in combination with other drugs, to lower blood pressure to normal with a minimum of side effects. In mild high blood pressure, your doctor may feel that a trial of dietary salt restriction is the first step to be taken. This is a complex decision, and there is no absolute right or wrong.

Drugs that lower blood pressure can act at a variety of different sites in the body. These include the brain, autonomic nervous system, nerve endings, heart and blood vessel "receptor sites," blood vessel walls, and, finally, the kidney itself. Most patients are first started on a diuretic or "water pill." These pills act to cause the kidney to excrete more sodium and thus result in a blood pressure drop.

The report of the Joint National Committee on Detection, Evaluation and Treatment of High Blood Pressure[33] makes six general recommendations on the treatment of high blood pressure:

1. Any group measuring blood pressure should have resources available for referral, confirmation and follow-up.
2. Virtually all patients with a diastolic (lower number) blood

pressure of 105 mm Hg. or greater should be treated with antihypertensive drug therapy.

3. For persons with diastolic pressure of 90–104 mm Hg. treatment should be individualized with consideration given to other risk factors.

4. The evaluation of patients with high blood pressure can be limited to a few baseline tests in most instances.

5. The stepped-care approach outline in this report is advocated as a cost-effective method of treating most patients.

6. Treatment of patients with high blood pressure includes plans for facilitating long-term maintenance of blood pressure controls.

The "stepped-care" approach to the treatment of high blood pressure has been advocated by the joint committees and is widely accepted. This regime recommends starting therapy with a small dose of an antihypertensive drug, increasing the dose of that drug, and, as necessary, adding one drug after another. This pyramiding of medication continues until effective control of the level of blood pressure is maintained. Periodic reevaluations allow for upward or downward titration of dosage schedules as required. There are many effective approaches to the therapy of high blood pressure, and in many cases therapy is individualized to the particular patient. Some of the more commonly used drugs to treat high blood pressure are summarized in Table 3-6.

The development of new, even more effective drugs continues. Physicians hope that these drugs will offer an advantage in lessening side effects while remaining effective. Drugs that specifically interfere with kidney enzymes (thought to play a role in high blood pressure) are being developed. The future looks bright with many new drugs in the offing.

YOU AND YOUR DOCTOR

Your doctor plays a vital role in your attempts to avoid the risks of high blood pressure. The condition is usually picked up on a routine physical examination. Elevations in blood pressure may or may not be deemed "significant" with the implications of lifelong treatment. This decision

TABLE 3-6. DRUGS COMMONLY USED TO TREAT HIGH BLOOD PRESSURE

Name	Dosage	Action	Contraindications and Side Effects	Comments
Chlorothiazide (Diuril)	250 mg 1000 mg every day	Diuretic (water pill)	Low blood potassium High blood sugar High blood uric acid (seen in gout) Rash	Blood chemistries to monitor potassium, sugar, and uric acid should be done.
Hydrochlorothiazide (Esidriz, Hydrodiuril, Oretic)	25 mg 100 mg every day	Diuretic (water pill)	Low blood potassium High blood sugar High blood uric acid Rash	Blood chemistries to monitor potassium, sugar, and uric acid should be done.
Chlorthalidone (Hygroton)	25 mg 100 mg every day	Diuretic (water pill)	Low blood potassium High blood sugar High blood uric acid Rash	Blood chemistries to monitor potassium, sugar, and uric acid should be done.
Methyclothiazide (Enduron)	2.5–5 mg every day	Diuretic (water pill)	Low blood potassium High blood sugar High blood uric acid Rash	Blood chemistries to monitor potassium, sugar, and uric acid should be done.
Hydroflumethiazide (Saluron)	50 mg every day	Diuretic (water pill)	Low blood potassium High blood sugar High blood uric acid Rash	Blood chemistries to monitor potassium, sugar, and uric acid should be done.
Furosemide (Lasix)	20–40 mg once a day or twice a day	Diuretic (water pill)	Low blood potassium High blood uric acid Diarrhea, nausea, and vomiting	Blood chemistries to monitor potassium and uric acid should be done.

(continued)

TABLE 3-6. (continued)

Name	Dosage	Action	Contraindications and Side Effects	Comments
Metolazone (Zaroxolyn)	2.5–5 mg every day	Diuretic (water pill)	Low blood potassium High blood sugar High blood uric acid	Blood chemistries to monitor potassium, sugar, and uric acid should be done.
Triamterene and hydrochlorothiazide (Dyazide)	1–2 capsules twice a day	Combination diuretic	Potassium imbalance High blood sugar High blood uric acid	Blood chemistries to monitor potassium, sugar, and uric acid should be done.
Propranolol hydrochloride (Inderal)	160–480 mg	Beta-blocking agent (blocks nerve stimulation—how this lowers blood pressure is *not* established)	This drug cannot be used in patients with asthma, heart failure, or slow heart rates.	Dosages of this drug have to be individualized according to blood pressure response.
Methyldopa (Aldomet)	500–2000 mg daily in divided doses	Lowers blood pressure, probably by direct effect on the central nervous system	Hepatitis Hemolytic anemia sedation, anxiety, diarrhea, impotence	Liver and blood tests should be monitored.
Prazosin hydrochloride (Minipres)	3–20 mg daily in divided doses	Direct effect on smooth muscle blood vessel walls	Dizziness, headache, drowsiness, weakness	Dose must be increased slowly and be individualized.

Drug	Dosage	Action	Side Effects	Comments
Clonidine hydrochloride (Catapres)	0.1–0.8 mg daily (maximum dosage 2.4 mg/day)	Direct central nervous system effect	Dry mouth, drowsiness, constipation, headache, fatigue	This drug should not be abruptly stopped, as it can cause nervousness, agitation, and headache.
Hydralazine hydrochloride (Apresoline)	40–200 mg daily in divided doses	Direct effect on smooth muscle of blood vessel walls	Headache, fast heart rate; cannot be used in patients with angina pectoris	With high dosages, irregular heart rates can be seen.
Chlorthalidone and reserpine (Regroton, Demi-Regroton)	1–2 tablets daily	Combination of diuretic and nerve ending action	Depression, peptic ulcer disease, low blood potassium, high blood sugar, high blood uric acid	This is an effective combination of two well-known drugs.
Metoprolol tartrate (Lopressor)	100 mg–450 mg daily in divided doses	Beta-blocking agent lowers blood pressure in a manner similar to propranolol	Slow heart rate, heart failure, asthma	Dosage of this drug has to be individualized according to blood pressure response. (This drug is somewhat more selective in its action as compared to propranolol.)

must be made by your doctor in light of his knowledge of you and your test results. The extent to which your doctor feels you need evaluation will vary from individual to individual. He may feel you only need a few screening tests or, on the other hand, an extensive evaluation (in the search for an underlying cause). Let us briefly discuss some of the tests he may obtain.

Urine

1. Urinalysis will give information about kidney function. The kidneys can be either a cause of high blood pressure or target organs for resulting damage. This test is simple but useful.
2. Twenty-four-hour urine for catecholamines, metanephrine, or vanillylmandelic acid. This test can give information about endocrine gland disorders that can cause high blood pressure.

Blood

1. Electrolytes. This blood test is important to establish a base-line value for sodium, potassium, chloride, and carbon dioxide in the blood and can also give a clue to other causes of high blood pressure.
2. Creatinine. This is a blood test useful as an indication of kidney function.
3. Fasting sugar. This is a blood test that is important to rule out other diseases, such as sugar diabetes, as well as establish a baseline priority to therapy.
4. Uric acid. This is a blood test useful in establishing the tendency toward gout since some types of hypertension treatment increase the risk of gout.
5. Cholesterol and triglycerides. This is a blood test important in establishing the extent of other risk factors of heart disease.

Electrocardiograms

The EKG is a graphic recording of the electrical activity of the heart during each beat. These electrical patterns or waves can be correlated with known disease states and abnormal situations. In addition, the EKG can give information about heart chamber size, an important measure in high blood pressure.

Chest X-ray

A chest x-ray can give information about the condition of your heart, lungs, and blood vessels in the chest. It allows for an accurate assessment of heart size, which is important in the diagnosis of high blood pressure.

Intravenous Pyelogram

This is an x-ray study of your kidneys. Dye is given in a vein and concentrated within the kidneys. This x-ray study reveals much information about the size and function of the kidney, which is important since kidney disease may be the cause of high blood pressure or result from its presence.

There are other studies that your doctor may need for his evaluation of you.

Remember, take high blood pressure seriously. You can lengthen your life by getting regular medical care and following your doctor's instructions. If high blood pressure runs in your family, cut down on your salt intake. You are not just a helpless victim of circumstance. Take control of those environmental factors that increase your risk and live longer.

REFERENCES

1. Stamler J: Cardiovascular disease in the United States. *American Journal of Cardiology* 10: 319–340, 1962.
2. Berkow R: *The Merck Manual of Diagnosis and Therapy.* Rahway, NJ, Merck Sharp & Dohme Research Labs, 1977, p. 388.
3. Kannel WB: Role of blood pressure in cardiovascular disease, the Framingham Study. *Angiology* 26: 1–14, 1975.
4. Freis E: Salt, volume and the prevention of hypertension. *Circulation* 53: 1976.
5. Oglesby P: Risks of mild hypertension: a ten-year report. *British Heart Journal* (Supple. 116–21), 1971.
6. Kannel WB: Role of blood pressure in cardiovascular disease, the Framingham Study. *Angiology* 26: 1–14, 1975.
7. Freis E, et al: VA Cooperative study group, effects of treatment on morbidity in hypertension. *JAMA* 213: 1145–52, 1970.
8. Freis E, et al: VA cooperative study group, effects of treatment on morbidity in hypertension. *JAMA* 202: 116–22, 1967.

9. Berglund G, et al: Coronary heart disease after treatment of hypertension. *Lancet* 1–5, 1978.

10. Detection, Evaluation and Treatment of High Blood Pressure. *USV Pharmaceutical Corp. Information Services.*

11. Freis E: Salt, volume and the prevention of hypertension. *Circulation*, 53: 1976.

12. Kawasaki T: The effect of high-sodium and low-sodium intakes on blood pressure and other related variables in human subjects with idiopathic hypertension. *American Journal of Medicine* 64: 193–98, 1978.

13. Gutman C, et al: Interaction of environmental factors and systemic arterial blood pressure: a review. *Medicine* Baltimore 59: 543–553, 1971.

14. Whitehead W, et al: Anxiety and anger in hypertension. *Journal of Psychiatric Research* 21: 383–89, 1977.

15. Meyer E, et al: Hypertension and psychological distress. *Psychosomatics* 160–68, 1978.

16. Heritability of blood pressure. *British Medical Journal* 127–38, 1978.

17. Heritability of blood pressure. *British Medical Journal* 127–38, 1978.

18. Kannel WB, et al: *Hypertension in Framingham, epidemiology and control of hypertension,* Paul O (ed). New York, Stratton Intercontinental Medical Corporation, 1978, pp. 553–92.

19. D'Alonza Ca, et al: Cardiovascular disease among problem drinkers, *Journal of Occupational Medicine* 10:344–50, 1968.

20. Klatsky A, et al: Alcohol consumption and blood pressure. *New England Journal of Medicine* 1194–99, 1977.

21. D'Alonza Ca, et al: Cardiovascular disease among problem drinkers, *Journal of Occupational Medicine* 10: 344–50, 1968.

22. Kannel WB, et al: The relation of adiposity to blood pressure and development of hypertension.

23. Chiang B, et al: Overweight & hypertension. *Circulation* 39: 402–21, 1969.

24. *Blood Pressure of Persons 18–74 years, United States, 1971–72.* National Health Survey, National Center for Health Statistics, Series II, 150. United States Department of Health, Education and Welfare, 1975.

25. McDonough JR, et al: Blood pressure and hypertensive disease among Negroes and whites. *Annals of Internal Medicine* 61: 208–28, 1964.

26. HDFP Cooperative Group, Original Contributions, Race Education and Prevalence of Hypertension. *American Journal of Epidemiology* 106: 351–361.

27. Acupuncture anesthesia: pricking the balloon. *JAMA* 237: 2530–31, 1977.

28. Kannel WB, et al: The relation of adiposity to blood pressure and development of hypertension.

29. Klatsky A, et al: Alcohol consumption and blood pressure. *New England Journal of Medicine* 1194–99, 1977.
30. Morgan T, et al: Hypertension Treated by Salt Restriction, *Lancet* 227–30, 1978.
31. Chiang B, et al: Overweight & hypertension, *Circulation* 39: 403–21, 1969.
32. Boyer J, et al: Exercise therapy in hypertensive men. *JAMA* 211: 1970.
33. Detection, Evaluation and Treatment of High Blood Pressure. *USV Pharmaceutical Corp. Information Services.*

FOUR

Blood Clot in the Lung

Blood clots in the lung (pulmonary embolism) will kill upwards of 200,000 people in the United States every year.[1] This health problem is the leading cause of death from lung disease in hospitalized patients.[2] Pulmonary embolism is also responsible for one out of every ten deaths after surgery.[3]

The disease was first described by Virchow in 1846, yet most of these deaths will go unrecognized as caused by blood clots in the lung until autopsy.[4] The tragedy of this is that had the diagnosis been made, many deaths could have been prevented.

Despite the widespread occurrence and common knowledge about pulmonary embolism, it often remains undetected. It is generally acknowledged that only a small fraction of these cases are diagnosed by the physician at the patient's side. Since there are protective measures that can be taken by your doctor, the sad result is that many more patients die from pulmonary embolism than might have. This particularly distressing fact has long been known by physicians, and there have been many suggestions for coping with the problem. An educated patient and an alert physician can prevent thousands of needless deaths. The large number of cases that are not diagnosed are not the result of "poor medical practice." Rather, it is the disease itself that has peculiarities that make diagnosis difficult.

Let's take a look at a few of the problems:

1. Blood clots in the lung (pulmonary emboli) are usually preceded by clots in the deep veins of the legs. If your doctor finds evidence of clots in your legs, there are steps he can take to protect you. Here's the catch. Most clots in the legs have no signs or symptoms clinically (although some do). In other words, no matter how astute your doctor is, most of these clots are clinically silent.

2. The signs and symptoms of blood clots in your lung are variable, inconsistent, and nonspecific. This is where the expertise and experience of your doctor is vital. For example, some cases of pulmonary embolism that are seen in emergency rooms are labeled "anxiety reactions." It takes real skill, a lot of experience, and a suspicious doctor to make the diagnosis.

3. Seventy to eighty percent of patients with fatal blood clots die within 1 to 2 hours after the onset of symptoms.[5] That does not give your physician enough time to do the more sophisticated tests to confirm the diagnosis.

Remember that the above are the problems. There are solutions; and you play a key part. As an educated patient, this chapter could save your life. Your physician has been working to improve the situation; as a result, there have been significant advances in medical thinking about pulmonary embolism. We'll talk about these changes in more detail later.

The brief list below represents conceptual changes in your doctor's thinking about pulmonary embolism. These are significant in that they form the backbone of a new attack on an old problem.[6]

1. The clinically silent nature of clots in the legs is now widely known, which not only leads to increased awareness by your doctor but also to the development of new diagnostic tools.

2. The importance of blood clots in the lung as a cause of death is

now accepted. For many years, its importance was grossly underestimated in official statistics, which was the result of technical difficulties during autopsy and most cases being undiagnosed clinically. Since its seriousness and extent have been widely underrated in the past, the problem was not attacked as vigorously as it is today.

3. Effective and safe prevention methods have been discovered. This exciting development has widespread potential benefit. The value of the protective measures is greatly enhanced when they can be used in people at higher risk.

4. The risk factors have been identified. In other words, we now know who is at greatest danger; therefore, physicians can key in to these specific patients and apply the prophylactic measures when needed.

Later in the chapter, we'll discuss what is currently known about risk and prevention. You'll learn if you're at risk and what can be done; quite literally, this could save your life. Remember you're an active participant in your medical care. Ask your doctor questions; it's your body. Unfortunately, not all physicians are completely aware of some of the information we'll discuss. In actuality, this is not a comment on your doctor's ability. It simply reflects the huge volume of information that exists and that no one person can reasonably be expected to know it all.

WHAT IS A BLOOD CLOT IN THE LUNG (PULMONARY EMBOLISM)?

More than 130 years ago, Virchow described occluding masses within the arteries supplying the lung. He was correct in suggesting that these blockages did not form locally but traveled through the blood stream until they lodged within a blood vessel and were unable to travel further. He theorized that these masses were actually clots formed in distant veins. These clots became dislodged and were carried by the blood to the heart and from there to the blood vessels supplying the lungs. It is in these blood vessels through which they can no longer pass that blood flow was blocked. Virchow was amazingly correct in his analysis.

In other words, pulmonary embolism is the lodgement of a blood clot in a pulmonary artery. These clots usually are first formed within the deep veins in the legs. Clots, also termed thrombi, break off and are carried through the blood stream to the pulmonary artery (the artery supplying the lung). Clots when formed in the veins of the leg are termed deep vein thromboses. The clot that may break off and travel to the lung originates frequently from the legs. Therefore, there is a direct relationship between a patient having deep vein thrombosis and his risk of a blood clot to the lung.

Blood clots to the lung sometimes originate in other veins. For example, they may come from veins in the pelvis (groin), abdomen, upper arms, or even the heart itself.

The clotting of blood is a normal and quite essential physiologic process that is vital to all our lives. It can be dangerous when these clots are "mistakenly" formed under certain conditions. We'll discuss those conditions later; in general, however, the key factors believed essential in forming these clots are:

1. Stasis — a change in blood flow rate and direction within the blood vessel.
2. Abnormalities in the blood vessel wall — damage, perhaps microscopic, to the blood vessel wall.
3. Alterations in the blood coagulation system — this means there is some inherent defect in the blood itself. This defect supposedly causes clots to form more readily (a popular notion but without much scientific support).

We've seen that a pulmonary embolism is simply a blood clot blocking a blood vessel to the lung. Why then is this so dangerous a situation? Let's take a closer look at the consequences of this event.[7]

Acute event

A blood clot lodges within a blood vessel supplying the lung. This effectively blocks the blood supply to the lung tissue beyond the obstruction. The loss of blood to the lung tissue involved varies with the size of the clot and/or the number of clots, which sets off a series of processes in the lung:

1. There is now an area of lung tissue that can take air in with breathing as it did before. However, the blood supply to that

lung has been cut off. It is in the blood that the carbon dioxide and oxygen are carried. Therefore, fresh oxygen taken into that lung area cannot enter the blood stream. Conversely, carbon dioxide cannot be blown off into the air. Therefore, the breathing or ventilation of that portion of the lung serves no purpose. This is termed "wasted ventilation."

2. The air sacs in the lung tissue stay open because of a chemical known as surfactant. Without surfactant, the lung will collapse. When the blood supply to an area of lung is cut off, levels of this chemical start to drop within 2 to 3 hours. This worsens with time, so that at 24 to 48 hours, there is frank collapse of the lung tissue involved.

3. The decline in blood supply to the lung can also lead to a failure in the heart's ability to pump blood, heart failure, and a rapid heart rate.

Since even small blood clots can cause a lot of problems, whether a pulmonary embolus is life threatening or minor depends on the size of the clot and, perhaps most importantly, the physical condition of the patient prior to the blood clot.

SIGNS AND SYMPTOMS OF PULMONARY EMBOLISM

As mentioned previously, the signs and symptoms that may suggest a pulmonary embolus are nonspecific and variable (Table 4-1).

TABLE 4-1. SIGNS AND SYMPTOMS OF PULMONARY EMBOLISM

Difficulty or distress in breathing, frequently rapid breathing (dyspnea)

Pain, usually sharp, upon taking a deep breath (pleuritic chest pain)

Anxiety

Coughing up blood (hemoptysis)

Chest pressurelike discomfort

Note: These are some of the signs and symptoms that may be present with a pulmonary embolism. Remember, they are not specific, do not all have to be present, and may indicate another ailment.

The most common complaint is a sudden feeling of difficulty breathing or being unable to catch your breath. Some patients will complain of feeling anxious. Still others may have sharp chest pain upon taking a deep breath or may cough up blood.

All of these symptoms and signs can be manifestations of another illness. There may be only one of these complaints or several. Your doctor must use his skill to evaluate your complaints in the light of laboratory evaluations, your exposure to known risk factors, physical examination, and, finally, his knowledge of you as an individual. Later in

TABLE 4-2. CONDITIONS ASSOCIATED WITH A HIGH RISK OF PULMONARY EMBOLISM

The period after surgery (This risk is greater in patients with other known risk factors, for example, cancer, obesity.)

Pregnancy: especially after delivery (infrequent but serious)

Ulcerative colitis

Birth control pills

Infections

Heart disease (especially heart failure or an abnormal heart rhythm known as atrial fibrillation)

Varicose veins or previous phlebitis

Chronic lung disease (emphysema, chronic bronchitis)

Obesity

Immobilization (eg, long automobile rides, after trauma)

Paralysis

Trauma (especially fractures or injuries to the legs or hips)

Advancing age

Poor blood vessel supply to the legs

Length of bed rest (risk increases with duration of bed rest)

Cancer (increased risk with all types; however, the risk varies with the specific type)

Previous episodes of deep vein thrombosis or pulmonary embolism

From Wintrobe.[4]

the chapter, we'll discuss the physical examination and the laboratory tests.

WHAT ARE THE RISK FACTORS FOR PULMONARY EMBOLISM?

This is a particularly important issue in pulmonary embolism. In the first place, there are prophylactic steps that can be applied to patients at high risk. Furthermore, in an extensive review[8,9] of all patients with pulmonary embolism as the cause of death, 50 percent would have been expected to live a considerable time had they not had a pulmonary embolism.[10]

When we talk about risk factors for pulmonary embolism, we must also examine the risk factors for deep vein thrombosis. Since deep vein thrombosis is a frequent precursor of pulmonary embolism, there is no logical consideration of one without the other.

There has been a great deal of research in this area. Table 4-2 summarizes those conditions known to have a high risk of pulmonary embolism. From a slightly different perspective, Table 4-3 shows us which groups of people are more likely to develop blood clots in the veins (deep vein thrombosis); remember, there is a direct relationship between deep vein thrombosis and pulmonary embolism.

In order to underscore the importance of risk factors in pulmonary embolism, remember that current medical treatment is directed at preventing their occurrence. Treatment of individuals at known higher risk extends the potential for prevention. Let's take a closer look at these risk factors:

TABLE 4-3. GROUPS ASSOCIATED WITH A HIGH INCIDENCE OF DEEP VEIN THROMBOSIS

Patients over the age of 40 with fractures of the lower extremities or hips, especially for whom a period of ten days or more of immobilization is anticipated
Patients with heart attacks, especially in the presence of other risk factors such as duration of bed rest and heart failure
Patients undergoing major abdominal, thoracic, or gynecologic surgery

From Wintrobe.[4]

Heart disease

Heart disease is a very important risk factor in the development of deep vein thrombosis and pulmonary embolism. In hospitalized patients, this has been well studied and is important both in total numbers and percentage of patients affected.[11,12] In an autopsy-proved pulmonary embolism study,[13] the average occurrence in people with heart disease, 30 years or older, was 20.4 percent. In those patients with heart failure, the frequency of pulmonary embolism rose to 27.5 percent and was an even higher 35.9 percent in the presence of the abnormal heart rhythm known as atrial fibrillation. The author concludes that any type of heart disease increases the chance of pulmonary embolism three times in patients over 30. The risk is even greater in heart failure or atrial fibrillation.

Heart attacks may be a risk factor independently. (Remember, heart attacks are a manifestation of underlying heart disease.) There is some debate about this. In one autopsy review, it was noted that there was no increase in pulmonary embolism in the group with heart attacks when compared with patients with the same underlying type of heart disease.[14] However, the same author notes that in patients with heart attacks, the incidence of deep vein thrombosis is 30 to 40 percent.[15] (Remember, deep vein thrombosis is the precursor of pulmonary emboli.) In a British review, the occurrence of deep vein thrombosis after a heart attack was thought to be related to the severity of the heart attack or the presence of heart failure.[16]

Cancer

Cancer was first associated with the development of clots more than 100 years ago. There is an increased incidence of deep vein thrombosis with all types of cancer. Cancer patients, as a group, have a two to three times greater chance of developing a pulmonary embolism.[17]

It's also known that different types of cancer carry with them increased risk and that this risk varies with the type of tumor. Cancer of the pancreas, for example, has the highest danger (almost six times greater than other types). Also at greater risk are patients with bladder-kidney (genitourinary) cancer, stomach cancer, colon (large bowel) cancer, and breast cancer[18] (Table 4-4).[19]

Patients who undergo surgery and have cancer have about 1.5

TABLE 4-4. RISK OF PULMONARY EMBOLISM IN PATIENTS WITH CANCER

Type of Cancer	Risk of Pulmonary Embolism (%)
Pancreas	35.1
Genitourinary (bladder-kidney)	20.6
Lung	20.1
Colon (large bowel)	18.7
Uterus, cervix (womb)	18.3
Prostate	16.7
Stomach	15.8
Breast	15.1
All others	8.4

From Coon.[1]
Note: In brief summary, the risk of pulmonary embolism in patients with cancer is threefold with breast cancer, genitourinary cancer, stomach cancer, colon and lung cancer and six times in patients with cancer of the pancreas.

times the risk of development of deep vein thrombosis as those people operated upon without cancer.[20] There have been many different explanations for this association between cancer and blood clots.

Changes in the blood clotting factors and blood constituents have been noted. None of these are proven to be the cause of the clots.

Obesity

After surgery, obese patients have an increased risk of deep vein thrombosis of 1.5 to 2 times the risk of normal-weight patients.[21] In a review of this increased risk of obese patients, the authors point out that there are several possible explanations for the increased risk of deep vein thrombosis and pulmonary emboli.[22] Obese patients have higher levels of plasma fatty acids and are less mobile as well. Both these factors may explain the increased risk. As we'll see later, decreased mobility is a risk factor for deep vein thrombosis independently.

The plasma fatty acids are thought to initiate the "cascade" of events that lead to blood clot formation. This can occur through either damage to the inside surface of the blood vessel walls or binding of fatty acids to these walls.

Whatever the mechanism, in one autopsy study, patients 20 percent overweight had a rate of pulmonary embolism of 21.9 percent.[23] This was a statistically significant increase in pulmonary emboli in the obese. There is a recent study in which extremely overweight patients underwent surgery to bypass their stomachs and thereby reduce weight. In that study, the authors concluded that these markedly obese patients were not at high risk from pulmonary embolism.[24] This study runs counter to most accepted evidence, that is, that obesity is generally acknowledged to be a risk factor in deep vein thrombosis and pulmonary embolism.

Accidental Trauma

In a review of the association of pulmonary embolism and trauma, the authors point out several interesting findings.[25] They noted 1 percent of patients admitted to the hospital with trauma have a fatal pulmonary embolism and all patients with injury are at increased risk of deep vein thrombosis or pulmonary embolism. This risk varies with the nature and site of the injury. As reported in this paper, the risk of pulmonary embolism rises as listed below:

- Head and chest injuries (2 to 5 percent)
- Burns (5 to 8 percent)
- Spinal (backbone) fractures (14 percent)
- Pelvic (hip) fractures (27 percent)
- Tibial and femoral (long bones of the legs) fractures (45 to 60 percent)

In other words, fractures (breaks) in the legs are the most frequent causes of fatal pulmonary embolism after trauma. The authors also note that the most common cause of death after hip fractures is felt to be pulmonary embolism. In one study, 38 percent and in another, 50 percent of the deaths in patients dying after hip fractures were caused by pulmonary emboli.

The authors also note that the risk of deep vein thrombosis from the trauma is not independent of surgery, if needed for treatment, and bed rest, both of which are known risk factors themselves.

Surgery

Surgery itself is most likely a risk factor. The risk of surgery is increased in the presence of other known risk factors. In a comprehensive review article,[26] patients aged 40 and over undergoing major operations have shown a 15 to 50 percent likelihood of developing deep vein thrombosis. Commenting further on the problem, the authors add that not all of these clots are believed to be at high risk of dislodging and becoming pulmonary emboli. It is thought that only the 10 to 30 percent of clots that extend into veins above the knee are associated with a high risk of pulmonary embolism.

The extent of surgery seems to correlate more with the risk of deep vein thrombosis or pulmonary embolism than does the site of surgery except in cases of trauma, as noted above. The explanation for this may be the immobilization or prolonged bed rest that may follow trauma-related surgery. Bed rest or immobility are risk factors. The longer the length of bed rest, the more likely the occurrence of deep vein thrombosis.

The authors remind us that the danger of thrombosis or pulmonary embolism after surgery varies with the presence of other risk factors. This increased risk can range from 50 percent in obese patients to 300 percent in patients with heart disease.

In summary, the risk of surgery increases with the amount of surgery, site of surgery (in trauma-related surgery), and presence of other risk factors. For example, the risk of deep vein thrombosis or pulmonary embolism after gall bladder is threefold greater than after a hernia repair.[27]

Age

There are several studies that conclude that there is an increasing risk of pulmonary embolism with age.[28,29] There are several plausible explanations for this. These include:

1. The known association of other diseases, including heart disease and cancer with advancing age.
2. Anatomic changes in the blood vessels of the lower limbs, which may lead to a slowing of blood flow "stasis" and therefore the formation of clots.
3. The relative immobility of the elderly and the greater duration

of bed rest after surgery. These factors are all linked to an increased formation of clots.

Pregnancy

Deep vein thrombosis was first linked to pregnancy in the eighteenth century. At the time, it was believed that these painful and swollen legs were caused by excess breast milk that was deposited in the legs. These were termed *"depots de lait"* and *"phlegmatia lactia"*; even recently deep vein thrombosis during pregnancy has been called "milk leg."[30]

The increased risk to women who are pregnant or post partum (after delivery) is more than five fold that of nonpregnant women not taking birth control pills.[31]

Deep vein thrombosis is the second most common cause of maternal death according to some reviews.[32,33] However, one study examining records during a ten-year period in two community hospitals concluded that pulmonary embolism was an infrequent but serious complication[34] in pregnancy. Estimates vary, but pulmonary embolism is probably responsible for 30 deaths in every million deliveries.

The risk factors that increase the danger to the pregnant woman include cesarean section, assisted delivery, the use of estrogens to decrease milk production, and older age of the pregnant women. The risk of fatal pulmonary embolism after section is nine times greater than by birth canal delivery.[35]

Pregnancy is a definite risk factor in pulmonary embolism and accounts for one-half of all thrombosis in pulmonary embolism in women under 40.[36]

Estrogens and Birth Control Pills

In a comparative review of estrogens and oral contraceptives, the authors report the following:[37]

1. Estrogens increase the risk of the development of deep vein thrombosis or pulmonary embolism. In British studies, the risk was increased sevenfold, whereas in a U.S. study the risk was estimated to be increased forty-four-fold.
2. Annual death rates in women using birth control pills were increased an estimated seven times. The elevated risk remains

constant as long as these pills are used and continues for several weeks after they are stopped.

3. There is an apparent correlation between the dose of estrogen in the pill and the risk.

4. Women given estrogens to lessen milk production are at three times greater risk of developing deep vein thrombosis or pulmonary embolism.

5. There is an increased risk in women of blood types A, AB, and B who are taking birth control pills.

6. Women taking birth control pills in the month before surgery or with trauma face a risk of pulmonary embolism or deep vein thrombosis that is four to six times higher. A British review of estrogen-containing birth control pills also notes the following:[38]

   a. Risk of hospitalization for deep vein thrombosis or pulmonary embolism is six to seven times higher among married women who use birth control pills.

   b. They also agree that the risk is related to estrogen dosage.

In summary, there does appear to be a risk associated with birth control pills. That risk is related to the amount of estrogen in the pill. In addition, the risk continues for several weeks after the pills are stopped.

Varicose veins

There are many studies that confirm that patients with varicose veins are at higher risk for deep vein thrombosis and pulmonary embolism. After surgery, patients with varicose veins have a two-to-threefold greater incidence of these problems.[39]

Previous Deep Vein Thrombosis or Pulmonary Embolism

Patients with a history of previous deep vein thrombosis have an increased risk after surgery. This increased risk has been noted by several authors and has been known for many years.[40,41] In one study, a 68.4 percent prevalence of deep vein thrombosis was found after surgery in patients who had a prior episode. Another study demonstrated a threefold greater increase in risk in postsurgery patients who had a previous episode.[42]

Ulcerative colitis

People with chronic ulcerative colitis have a risk increased two-to-threefold of developing deep vein thrombosis or pulmonary embolism. A possible explanation for this is the blood-clotting abnormalities reported in this disease.[43]

Paralysis and immobility

Paralyzed and immobilized patients have an increased risk of deep vein thrombosis and pulmonary embolism. This varies with the duration of bed rest in hospitalized patients. It has also been reported in rather unique situations.[44] For example, fatal pulmonary embolism was noted to be increased in elderly patients confined to chairs in air raid shelters during World War II. It has also been seen in people after long automobile or airplane rides or prolonged sitting for other reasons. An autopsy study shows a rapid rise in the frequency of venous thrombosis that begins within 3 days of the start of bed rest. It rises to 15 percent in patients who have been confined to bed for up to 7 days and reaches 90 percent in people confined between 3 and 4 weeks.[45]

TABLE 4-5. POSSIBLE RISK FACTORS IN PULMONARY EMBOLISM

Nutritional factors

Alcohol

Arthritis

Hyperlipidemia (elevated levels of fat in the blood)

Variations in degree of physical activity

Drugs (other than birth control pills and estrogens)

Steroids

Several antibiotics

E aminocaproic acid

Blood type (A, increased risk; O, decreased risk)

Diabetes mellitus (sugar diabetes)

Heart attacks

Crohn's disease

There are other factors that are not definitely proved but are suspected to be risk factors for deep vein thrombosis and pulmonary embolism (Table 4-5 and 4-6).

TABLE 4-6. NOT A RISK FACTOR FOR PULMONARY EMBOLISM

Smoking habits

Social class

Race

Sex (in hospitalized patients): in a community study, females had a tenfold greater frequency of vein thrombosis. One-half of these related to pregnancy.

Risk factors are especially important in pulmonary embolism since there are many lives lost, and there is effective prophylactic treatment that can be given by your doctor. Such treatment cannot reasonably be given to everyone undergoing hospitalization. The ability to recognize those people at high risk should allow your doctor to protect selectively those individuals to some degree.

Remember, earlier we said that it is estimated one-half of obese patients would have been expected to have survived for a considerable period had pulmonary embolism not caused their death.

WHAT YOU CAN DO ABOUT PULMONARY EMBOLISM

There are definite steps that can be taken. Most of the prevention in the form of prophylactic drugs has to be administered by your physician. Take an active role in your medical care. Look at the risk factors as we've discussed them. If surgery or hospitalization is anticipated for yourself or a family member, see if any of the risk factors are present. If they are, ask your doctor about prevention (we'll discuss this later) and whether he or she feels it appropriate (Table 4-7).

There are several things you can do yourself. Probably the most important one you've already taken by learning the risk factors. The others are simple (Table 4-8):

- If you're overweight, go on a reasonable diet with the help of your doctor. Avoid "fad" diets, which may be dangerous. Diet is especially important if elective surgery is planned. Lose weight first; it may save your life.
- Avoid prolonged bed rest or long periods of immobility. If you are ill, get out of bed as soon as possible (unless it's inappropriate, according to your doctor).
- If you're taking birth control pills, stop them at least 1 month before any elective surgery. As we've seen, they not only increase your risk but continue to keep you at higher risk for a few weeks after they're stopped.

Treatment of Pulmonary Embolism

After the diagnosis of pulmonary embolism has been made, the medical management is determined by two factors:[46]

TABLE 4-7. WHAT CAN BE DONE TO LESSEN THE RISK OF PULMONARY EMBOLISM

Small doses of blood-thinning medication given to groups at higher risk (mini-dose heparin)

Elastic stockings or bandages in situations requiring prolonged bed rest

Early ambulation in post-partum and postoperative periods (after delivery and after surgery)

Intermittent calf compression

Elevation of the affected leg

Utilization of new techniques for increasing detection of blood clots in the veins (deep vein thrombosis) thus allowing for preventive measures, such as the above, to be utilized in this group of people who are at higher risk

TABLE 4-8. WHAT YOU CAN DO TO LESSEN YOUR RISK

Lose weight, especially prior to elective surgery.

Avoid long periods of immobilization, including long automobile or plane trips.

Stop taking birth control pills at least one month prior to elective surgery.

1. The extent of damage done by the blood clot(s) to the circulatory system of the body.
2. The knowledge that in time most clots will resolve. Therefore, therapy is directed toward sustaining life until resolution occurs and preventing further clots from dislodging and going to the lung.

In other words, in cases in which the pulmonary embolism is not fatal and the patient survives the initial episode, the aim of therapy is to prevent another episode and support the patient.

The prevention of another embolism can most often be accomplished by medical therapy with an anticoagulant (blood thinner). The blood thinner helps prevent the formation of clots. Heparin is the drug of choice for several reasons:[47]

1. Its immediate onset of action.
2. It is very effective in stopping blood clotting formation.
3. It may help dissolve already-formed clots and
4. Its action can be rapidly reversed (in cases in which there may be the danger of, or actual, bleeding).

There are several different dosages and ways in which heparin can be given. It can be given either intermittently or by continuous administration through a vein. It can also be given in an injection under the skin. It is also recommended that the patient have bed rest for at least 5 to 7 days (since that's the time it takes for clots to become firmly attached to the nasal wall).

The oral blood thinners, for example, coumadin, are not recommended for initial therapy. Their main utilization is in preventing blood clots from forming for a prolonged period. This is used in situations in which the danger of a recurrence is high, that is, the presence of risk factors like heart failure, prolonged bed rest, etc., are present.

Surgical treatment for pulmonary embolism does exist, but it is seldom used. It is only felt useful (1) if the patient is so critically ill he cannot await medical therapy and (2) if the patient has a blood disorder that causes bleeding.

There are two different types of surgery possible. The first involves interrupting the major veins (through which the clots travel to the lungs). The second is surgically removing the clot from the lungs.

The first approach is an attempt to "block" the clots (within the major vein draining the lower part of the body: the inferior vena cava) before they reach the lung. There are many different techniques, both surgical and nonsurgical. It is currently believed that these techniques are not effective in preventing especially long-term recurrences of blood clots. Therefore, many feel that interruption of the inferior vena cava should be considered a *lifesaving procedure* to be used only in patients who could not tolerate an immediate recurrence of pulmonary emboli.[48]

The alternative surgical technique is to remove surgically the clot from the lungs (pulmonary embolectomy). This surgery is reported to have a 50 percent mortality associated with it. It is rarely used and should only be considered in patients who are in severe distress.

NEW FRONTIERS

Prevention is the real objective in the treatment of pulmonary embolism. There are some very exciting developments in this area. These new discoveries are making prevention a real possibility:

1. There are now improved methods to allow early detection of deep vein thrombosis (the precursor of pulmonary embolism). These techniques, therefore, could be used to determine early clots and allow for the use of preventive measures.
2. The risk factors are known in pulmonary embolism and deep vein thrombosis. Therefore, we also know who is most likely at increased risk.
3. The effectiveness of prophylactic therapy, "mini-dose heparin," starting prior to surgery has been demonstrated in many studies.[49,50] One of these, an international multicenter study with 4121 patients over 40 who underwent surgery, shows low-dose heparin is effective in the prevention of fatal postsurgical emboli.

Earlier we noted that most cases of pulmonary embolism and deep vein thrombosis are not diagnosed at the bedside. We stated that in those people who died from pulmonary embolism, one-half would have been expected to have survived for a considerable period. We also saw that 200,000 people in the United States will die of pulmonary emboli.

Considering the above, the implications of these new developments may someday potentially save thousands of lives.

YOU AND YOUR DOCTOR

Your physician plays an important role in protecting you from the dangers of pulmonary embolism. Since we said that only a fraction of cases were diagnosed at the bedside, you're probably concerned about that. Let's take a look at the way your doctor approaches the problem. The most consistent symptom associated with pulmonary embolism is breathlessness. There may or may not be coughing up of blood, chest pain, and anxiety. The symptoms and signs are variable.

The physical examination may be relatively normal.[51] There may be a few "noises" in the lungs but not necessarily. The most consistent finding on examination of the heart is a rapid heart rate. Examination of the legs and determining that deep vein thrombosis (or phlebitis) is present are very helpful. However, less than one-half the patients with pulmonary embolism have clinical evidence of clots in the leg veins. (Clots can come from places other than leg veins. Even when they come from leg veins, they may not be clinically detectable.) Body temperature is usually normal. From the above, it should be clear that from examination and symptoms alone, your doctor can at best suspect the correct diagnosis. He then must proceed to laboratory studies.

Lab studies that are routinely obtained are often not very helpful.

Complete blood count (CBC). This yields little or no information toward the correct diagnosis.

Blood chemistries. This blood test[52] yields little definitive support toward the correct diagnosis. There is a so-called "diagnostic triad" of increased serum bilirubin, increased serum lactic dehydrogenase (LDH), and normal serum glutamic oxaloacetic transaminase (SGOT) that actually is of little value.

Electrocardiogram (EKG). This tracing of your heart's electrical activity may show a fast heart rate but is otherwise normal in most patients. There may be other changes when there are many blood clots lodged in the lungs.

Chest x-ray. There may be positive findings on chest x-ray with pulmonary embolism. There may be infiltrates (LoLite densities) seen on the x-ray film. Other findings noted are subtle and include differences in size of the right and left pulmonary arteries and tapering of the blood vessels or areas of the lung that appear darker (radiolucenary) because of decreased blood flow. *Many people with pulmonary embolism have normal chest x-rays.*

Fluoroscopy. This is an x-ray study. A blood vessel in the lung will have fewer or no pulsations. Fluoroscopy can be helpful to the diagnosis, but it is not frequently used.

Arterial blood gasses. This is a blood test that measures the oxygen and carbon dioxide in your arterial blood. This blood test is different from the usual in that the blood must be gotten from an artery (usually the wrist, inner elbow, or groin). With pulmonary embolization, this test is helpful. Often, there is seen a low arterial oxygen and carbon dioxide level as well as more alkaline blood (arterial hypoxemia, hypocapnia, and respiratory alkalosis).

All the above tests can be normal and are not very specific. At this point your doctor may proceed to either one or both of two more specific studies:

The lung scan (photoscans, pulmonary perfusion, scintiphotography). Lung scans are images of the lung obtained by radioactive particles that show the distribution of pulmonary blood flow. These particles are injected into the veins; as they pass into the lungs, they emit gamma particles. The radioactive material injected is most often albumen labeled with iodine-131 or technetium-99. The particles are trapped in the small blood vessels of the lung. After they are injected, a detectory device records the patterns that are emitted. Normal scans show a smooth distribution of radioactivity and a pattern consistent with the normal anatomy of the lungs.

Uneven or absent radioactivity in an area indicates that there is abnormal blood flow to that area. Areas with absent or decreased radioactivity give a great deal of evidence toward the diagnosis of pulmonary embolism. The procedure is "simple, safe, and rapid."

It is not specific for pulmonary embolism since other diseases can give abnormal distribution of blood flow. For example, pneumonia, collapsed lung, emphysema, sarcoidosis, tuberculosis, etc, can all produce defects. For this reason, it is sometimes coupled with a ventilation study. In other words, a radioactive gas like Xc-133 is inhaled. This ventilation study gives information on where the air goes in your lung. Together, these two give much more specific evidence for pulmonary embolism. If the ventilation to an area is normal but the blood supply has been cut off, then pulmonary embolism is a likely diagnosis.

Pulmonary angiography. Angiography involves the injection of dye (radiopaque material) through a tube advanced through the heart into the pulmonary artery. It gives direct visual pictures of the lung blood vessels. However, the procedure is invasive and entails risk and necessitates specially trained personnel. In addition, there is the possibility of errors of interpretation because of technique, injection artifacts, and an inability to evaluate the small blood vessels. In this study, as in the lung scan, a decrease in filling suggests pulmonary embolism.

It should be made clear at this point why the diagnosis can be so frequently missed. A very interesting study was done analyzing how a diagnosis was made in 60 patients with suspected pulmonary embolism.[53] These patients had clinical examinations, chest x-rays, and lung scans. Later, the scans and chest x-rays were reread. The results showed there was poor agreement between the first and second scan readings. Also, the chest x-rays didn't correlate with the clinical and scan assessments.

With the newer screening techniques for deep vein thrombosis, more widespread medical information about the risk factors for pulmonary embolism, and the evidence in support of prophylactic therapy in high-risk groups, there may be the basis for a promising new attack upon an old problem.

REFERENCES

1. Coon W: Epidemiology of venous thromboembolism. *Annals of Surgery* 1977.
2. Coon W: Risk factors in pulmonary embolism. *Surgery, Gynecology and Obstetrics* 143: 1976.
3. Verstraete M: The prevention of postoperative deep vein thrombosis and pulmonary embolism with low dose subcutaneous heparin and dextran. *Surgery, Gynecology and Obstetrics* 143: 1976.
4. Wintrobe MM, et al (eds): *Principles of Internal Medicine*, ed. 8. New York, McGraw-Hill, 1977.
5. Coon W: Risk factors in pulmonary embolism. *Surgery, Gynecology and Obstetrics* 143: 1976.
6. Morris G, et al: The aetiology of acute pulmonary embolism and the identification of high risk groups. *British Journal of Hospital Medicine*, 1977.
7. Wintrobe MM, et al (eds): *Principles of Internal Medicine*, ed. 8. New York, McGraw-Hill, 1977.

8. Verstraete M: The prevention of postoperative deep vein thrombosis and pulmonary embolism with low dose subcutaneous heparin and dextran. *Surgery, Gynecology and Obstetrics* 143: 1976.
9. Bissell S: Pulmonary thromboembolism associated with gynecologic surgery and pregnancy. American Journal of Obstetrics and Gynecology, 1977.
10. Coon W: Epidemiology of venous thromboembolism. *Annals of Surgery* 1977.
11. Coon W: Epidemiology of venous thromboembolism. *Annals of Surgery* 1977.
12. Coon W: Risk factors in pulmonary embolism. *Surgery, Gynecology and Obstetrics* 143: 1976.
13. Coon W: Risk factors in pulmonary embolism. *Surgery, Gynecology and Obstetrics* 143: 1976.
14. Coon W: Risk factors in pulmonary embolism. *Surgery, Gynecology and Obstetrics* 143: 1976.
15. Coon W: Epidemiology of venous thromboembolism. *Annals of Surgery* 1977.
16. Morris G, et al: The aetiology of acute pulmonary embolism and the identification of high risk groups. *British Journal of Hospital Medicine,* 1977.
17. Coon W: Epidemiology of venous thromboembolism. *Annals of Surgery* 1977.
18. Coon W: Epidemiology of venous thromboembolism. *Annals of Surgery* 1977.
19. Coon W: Risk factors in pulmonary embolism. *Surgery, Gynecology and Obstetrics* 143: 1976.
20. Coon W: Risk factors in pulmonary embolism. *Surgery, Gynecology and Obstetrics* 143: 1976.
21. Coon W: Epidemiology of venous thromboembolism. *Annals of Surgery* 1977.
22. Strauss R, et al: Operative risks of obesity. Surgery, Gynecology and Obstetrics, 146: 1978.
23. Coon W: Risk factors in pulmonary embolism. *Surgery, Gynecology and Obstetrics* 143: 1976.
24. Printen K, et al: Venous thromboembolism in the morbidly obese. *Surgery, Gynecology and Obstetrics* 147: 117, 1978.
25. Coon W: Epidemiology of venous thromboembolism. *Annals of Surgery* 1977.
26. Coon W: Risk factors in pulmonary embolism. *Surgery, Gynecology and Obstetrics* 143: 1976.
27. Morris G, et al: The aetiology of acute pulmonary embolism and the

identification of high risk groups. *British Journal of Hospital Medicine,* 1977.

28. Coon W: Epidemiology of venous thromboembolism. *Annals of Surgery* 1977.

29. Morris G, et al: The aetiology of acute pulmonary embolism and the identification of high risk groups. *British Journal of Hospital Medicine,* 1977.

30. Morris G, et al: The aetiology of acute pulmonary embolism and the identification of high risk groups. *British Journal of Hospital Medicine,* 1977.

31. Coon W: Epidemiology of venous thromboembolism. *Annals of Surgery* 1977.

32. Coon W: Epidemiology of venous thromboembolism. *Annals of Surgery* 1977.

33. Morris G, et al: The aetiology of acute pulmonary embolism and the identification of high risk groups. *British Journal of Hospital Medicine,* 1977.

34. Bissell S: Pulmonary thromboembolism associated with gynecologic surgery and pregnancy. *American Journal of Obstetric Gynecology,* 1977.

35. Morris G, et al: The aetiology of acute pulmonary embolism and the identification of high risk groups. *British Journal of Hospital Medicine,* 1977.

36. Coon W: Epidemiology of venous thromboembolism. *Annals of Surgery* 1977.

37. Coon W: Epidemiology of venous thromboembolism. *Annals of Surgery* 1977.

38. Morris G, et al: The aetiology of acute pulmonary embolism and the identification of high risk groups. *British Journal of Hospital Medicine,* 1977.

39. Coon W: Epidemiology of venous thromboembolism. *Annals of Surgery* 1977.

40. Kesley J, et al: Prediction of thromboembolism following total hip replacement. *Clinical Orthopaedics and Related Research* 114: 1976.

41. Morris G, et al: The aetiology of acute pulmonary embolism and the identification of high risk groups. *British Journal of Hospital Medicine,* 1977.

42. Coon W: Epidemiology of venous thromboembolism. *Annals of Surgery* 1977.

43. Coon W: Epidemiology of venous thromboembolism. *Annals of Surgery* 1977.

44. Coon W: Epidemiology of venous thromboembolism. *Annals of Surgery* 1977.
45. Morris G, et al: The aetiology of acute pulmonary embolism and the identification of high risk groups. *British Journal of Hospital Medicine*, 1977.
46. Wintrobe MM, et al (eds): *Principles of Internal Medicine*, ed. 8. New York, McGraw-Hill, 1977.
47. Wintrobe MM, et al (eds): *Principles of Internal Medicine*, ed. 8. New York, McGraw-Hill, 1977.
48. Wintrobe MM, et al (eds): *Principles of Internal Medicine*, ed. 8. New York, McGraw-Hill, 1977.
49. Bissell S: Pulmonary thromboembolism associated with gynecologic surgery and pregnancy. *American Journal of Obstetrics and Gynecology*, 1977.
50. Verstraete M: The prevention of postoperative deep vein thrombosis and pulmonary embolism with low dose subcutaneous heparin and dextran. *Surgery, Gynecology and Obstetrics* 143: 1976.
51. Wintrobe MM, et al (eds): *Principles of Internal Medicine*, ed. 8. New York, McGraw-Hill, 1977.
52. Wintrobe MM, et al (eds): *Principles of Internal Medicine*, ed. 8. New York, McGraw-Hill, 1977.
53. Diagnostic decision-process in suspected pulmonary embolism. *Lancet*, 1979.

FIVE

Breast Cancer

In the United States, breast cancer ranks as the most deadly form of cancer in women.[1] It remains the most common cancer American women develop. The disease is the leading cause of death in women aged 35 to 54[2] and in subsequent years ranks second only to heart disease.

The serious extent of the public health problem breast cancer poses is further underscored by available statistics. It is estimated that this year 109,000 new cases of this cancer will be found and that more than 36,000 deaths will result. Nearly 1 out of every 11 women in the United States will develop breast cancer during her lifetime.[3]

Despite many new developments in treatment and early screening techniques, breast cancer continues unabated as a cause of death and infirmity. As a result, major efforts have turned toward the identification of risk factors in breast cancer in an attempt aimed at eventual prevention. During the past 15 years, intensive study has yielded an enormous body of knowledge.[4] However, the determination of the factors common to the development of breast cancer remains a goal for future continued and increased study.

WHAT IS BREAST CANCER?

Breast cancer is a disease characterized by the conversion of normal cells found in the breast into malignant cells. These cells are different from the normal cells in several important ways. Although most normal cells have the ability to reproduce themselves, malignant cells no longer retain the cellular mechanisms to control this replication. In other words, they multiply in a wild and uncontrolled fashion. With time and continued replication, these cells can cluster together and form a mass or tumor.

Nonmalignant cells may also cluster and form a tumor. In this situation, they represent no danger and are aptly termed benign tumors. Most breast masses found by the patient are benign.

Tumors comprised of malignant cells are known as malignant tumors. A malignant tumor in the breast is more specifically termed breast cancer.

Breast cancer cells, unlike benign cells, have the ability to invade and destroy neighboring normal tissue. By a process known as metastasis, tumor cells can break away and spread to other parts of the body. Upon spread of tumor cells to other areas of the body, the cells may implant and continue to replicate. In this way, new tumor masses may be produced. Eventually, the tumor growth may endanger the life of the patient. Breast cancer cells have a predilection for spread to particular areas of the body (Table 5-1).

TABLE 5-1. MOST LIKELY AREAS TO WHICH BREAST CANCER MAY SPREAD (METASTASIZE)

Lymph nodes (lymph glands)

Bone

Lung

Liver

Skin

Brain

Most cases of breast cancer are discovered by the patient herself when she feels a painless mass in the breast.[1] Less often, the mass is found by a physician or at a screening evaluation. It is generally accepted that the earlier a breast cancer is found, the better the patient's chances for prolonged life or cure.

Therefore, it becomes important for the patient to practice breast self-examination and to know the signs and symptoms of breast cancer

TABLE 5-2. BREAST SELF-EXAMINATION

The American Cancer Society offers these excellent instructions on how to do breast self-examination. I have reprinted them for your information:

1. In the shower
   Examine your breasts during baths or showers; hands glide more easily over wet skin. Fingers flat, move gently over every part of each breast. Use right hand to examine left breast, left hand for right breast. Check for any lump, hard knot, or thickening.
2. Before a mirror
   Inspect your breasts with arms at your sides. Next, raise your arms high overhead. Look for any changes in contour of each breast: a swelling, dimpling of skin, or changes in the nipple. Then rest palms on hips and press down firmly to flex your chest muscles. Left and right breast will not exactly match—few women's breasts do.
3. Lying down
   To examine your right breast, pull a pillow or folded towel under your right shoulder. Place right hand behind your head. This distributes breast tissue more evenly on the chest. With the left hand, fingers flat, press gently in small circular motions around an imaginary clock face. Begin at the outermost top of your right breast for 12 o'clock, then move to 1 o'clock; and so on around the circle back to 12. A ridge of firm tissue in the lower curve of each breast is normal. Then move in an inch, toward the nipple; keep circling to examine every part of your breast, including the nipple. This requires at least three more circles. Now slowly repeat the procedure on your left breast with a pillow under your shoulder and left hand behind your head. Notice how your breast structure feels.
   Finally, squeeze the nipple of each breast gently between thumb and index finger. Any discharge, clean or bloody, should be reported to your doctor immediately. Remember, breast self-examination is the single most important thing you can do to protect yourself.

(Tables 5-2 and 5-3). Upon the discovery of any of these signs or symptoms, the advice of a physician should be sought without delay.

TABLE 5-3. SIGNS AND SYMPTOMS OF BREAST CANCER

Lump or thickening in the breast

Nipple discharge

Dimpling of the skin

Changes in the nipple shape

Pain or tenderness

Ulceration of the skin

Swelling of the skin

WHAT ARE THE RISK FACTORS FOR BREAST CANCER?

Breast cancer is a serious and worldwide health problem. Thus far, only limited success has accompanied advances in therapy and screening. Intensive study during the last decade has yielded a great deal of information about common risk factors and theoretical causes of breast cancer.

Determining the risk factors in breast cancer offers the hopeful promise of modifying those factors and preventing a disease that is a major killer in the world. The risk literature on breast cancer is both complex and frequently contradictory. However, some studies appear to be particularly solid and reliable, and those are the ones we will look at in more detail.

HAIR DYE USE AND BREAST CANCER

The possible relationship between the use of permanent hair dye and the risk of developing breast cancer has been the subject of several recent investigations. These studies were undertaken for the following reasons:

1. A study in 1978 demonstrated an excess of chromosomal changes in the white blood cells of women with dyed hair.[53]

2. Various components of hair dyes were found to cause cancer when fed in high doses to laboratory animals.[54]

3. Approximately 20 million Americans, mostly women, use hair dye each year.[5]

The size of the exposed population and the possibly incriminating laboratory and animal data made it a priority to study any possible increased risk of developing breast cancer associated with hair dye use.

Recently, a survey of 120,557 women aged 30 to 55 demonstrated a relationship between breast cancer and permanent hair dye use.[6] Confirming this result, a Canadian case-control study showed no increased risk of breast cancer in users of permanent hair dyes.[7]

A third study demonstrated no overall association between hair dye use and breast cancer. However, this study suggests a possible increased risk in women with benign breast disease who also use hair dyes.[8] The number of cases was too small to view the findings as conclusive. The authors noted this and called for further studies.

Thus, despite some initially ominous reports, it now appears probable that hair dye is not a risk factor for breast cancer.

VIRUSES AND BREAST CANCER

The possibility of a human virus causing or participating in the development of breast cancer has been seriously considered. The isolation of different cancer-causing viruses such as the Murine mammary tumor virus in mice and the Mason-Pfizer virus in the rhesus monkey has fueled speculation in this direction.

A recent review article in the journal *Cancer* examined the role of viruses in humans.[9] The author finds little evidence to support the idea that a virus actually causes breast cancer in humans. The possible transmission of such a virus from mother to daughter via breast milk is also discounted. Furthermore, the author points out that while it was once thought that some human milk contains particles similar to the cancer-causing viruses, such a thesis is now thought to be in error; such particles bear no relationship to the risk of breast cancer.

The report of a group of 19 experts on breast cancer risk who recently met in England also commented on the possible role of viruses in human breast cancer.[10] The report concluded that "there is no good evidence that a virus transmitted from one case to another has a role in human breast cancer."

Another review from Belgium notes that a virus is still a possibility as a causative agent in humans.[11] In view of the hypothesized transmission of this virus in the breast milk of nursing mothers, the author asks a very intriguing question: "If breast feeding is an important route of transmission, one could reasonably ask why the marked reduction of breast feeding in the Western world has not been accompanied by a decrease in the incidence of breast cancer."

The available evidence points less to a viral causation of human breast cancer than once thought; the question is still considered open.

ZINC, COPPER, AND BREAST CANCER

Trace elements such as zinc and copper have been associated with various cancers. Low levels of zinc in blood, high levels of copper, and the ratio of zinc to copper have been reported to be useful indicators of activity, extent of disease, and prognosis in a variety of tumors.[12] A recent study in which 80 patients with breast disease were evaluated prior to surgery took place at Memorial Sloan-Kettering Cancer Center.[13] This study attempted to show any relationship that might exist between zinc, copper, and breast cancer. No relationship was found among these parameters and either breast cancer or benign breast disease. The authors note that the low zinc seen in other studies is probably related to poor nutrition, and the reported relationship of zinc and copper to breast cancer may be spurious. Again, this is another initially suspicious area that now seems not to be a risk.

DIET, OBESITY, AND BREAST CANCER

After three "false alarms," we now come to an area that seems to increase the risk of breast cancer. It is becoming increasingly evident that both total dietary fat intake and obesity are major risk factors in the development of breast cancer. Further evidence suggests that obesity and the combination of obesity and cholesterol are not only risk factors for the initial development of breast cancer but that once breast cancer is present, they significantly reduce survival.[14]

The importance of dietary fat intake has been shown by data gathered from a multitude of sources. These include studies of international variation in breast cancer rates, case-control studies, analyses of migrant populations, changes that occur within a country as it becomes "Westernized," and laboratory research. All of the evidence points both to total dietary fat and obesity as significant risk factors in breast cancer.

A closer look at some of these studies will help illustrate and underscore the role of diet in breast cancer.

Both the incidence and the death rates for breast cancer show a marked worldwide variation, being higher in industralized countries. In one project, the rates of breast cancer in 34 countries were compared to patterns of individual food intake. Five major types of food substances were examined: animal protein, eggs, meat, sugar, and total fats. After controlling for confounding variables, this study showed that breast cancer incidence and death rates correlated well with animal protein and total dietary fat intake.[15] In other words, women who consume high quantities of meat and total fat tended to develop breast cancer more frequently than women with other eating patterns.

Let us look at one prominent example. Although breast cancer is the most common cancer among American women, in Japan it ranks third, cancer of the stomach and uterus being more prevalent. Against this background of a low incidence of breast cancer, a sharp rise in incidence in Japan has been noted since 1966. This correlates directly with a marked change in dietary habits in Japanese women. During the past 15 years, there has been an increase of more than 250 percent in dietary fat intake (mostly due to increased pork consumption). By comparison, the incidence of breast cancer in the United States has not significantly changed since 1930.[16]

Furthermore, an analysis of Japanese women who migrated to the United States gives more credence to the effect of environment (diet, socioeconomic level, "Westernization") on breast cancer incidence rates. The incidence of breast cancer in the period 1969 through 1971 among first-generation Japanese immigrants aged 35 to 64 years and living in San Francisco rose to a level almost three times that of native Japanese women. In a similar pattern, Japanese Americans (the offspring of the first-generation immigrants) have a breast cancer rate approaching that of white American women.[17]

Laboratory evidence also supports the role of dietary fat in the etiology of breast cancer. An excellent review of dietary factors and breast cancer summarizes this data.[18] As early as 1942, it was suggested that a high fat diet enhances the rate of breast cancer development in laboratory animals. More recent studies have confirmed this early finding.

A more recent study confirms earlier reports of the significance of cholesterol and obesity in the prognosis of patients with breast cancer.[19] Of 374 patients with surgically treated breast cancer, those patients who were overweight prior to surgery had significantly poorer 5-year survivals. Patients who were both overweight and had high serum cholesterol levels had the worst 5-year survivals (32 percent) when compared to the normal weight and normal cholesterol group.

It is apparent from these data and a great many other studies that dietary fat intake and obesity are both important risk factors in breast cancer. It is also becoming evident that these factors decrease survival in patients with already diagnosed breast cancer.

The mechanism of action of dietary fat on the risk of breast cancer development is not definitively known. The most common theory concerns the apparent ability of fatty tissue in the body to synthesize the family of female hormones called estrogens. In particular, the naturally occurring estrogen known as estrone is a suspected culprit. However, there are a multitude of theories regarding the role of hormones in the development of breast cancer. Another common hormonal theory has to do with the role of so-called unopposed estrogens in breast tissue stimulation. This hormonal state is one in which there are high estrogen levels and low levels of progesterone, a different hormone. This situation naturally occurs in the premenopausal period and in the period from prepuberty to the delivery of the first full-term pregnancy.

RADIATION AND BREAST CANCER

Available data indicate that the breast is the organ most sensitive to radiation-induced cancer. Females aged 10 to 19 are more susceptible to these radiation-related changes than their older counterparts. Excess risk is reported to be directly proportional to the radiation dose received in the higher dose ranges of radiation exposure. Also, the effect of radiation appears to be cumulative, that is, individuals who receive the same total dose of radiation in repeated lower-dose exposures are not at reduced risk.[20,21]

The determination of risk from low-dose exposure is based on theoretical calculations. Data obtained from women previously exposed to high-dose radiation have been analyzed and revealed a linear dose-response relationship. In other words, the greater the radiation exposure, the more likely is a woman to develop breast cancer.

These data were obtained from women who were survivors at Hiroshima and Nagasaki, women who underwent multiple flouroscopies while being treated in a Nova Scotia tuberculosis sanitorium and women with mastitis (a benign breast inflammation) previously treated with radiation therapy. From this information, it has been theoretically postulated that if 1 million women received a single low-dose breast exposure of 1 rad of radiation, three to eight would develop breast cancer each year after a latent period of 10 to 20 years.[22] It is important to note, however, that no direct evidence of excess breast cancer risk has ever been seen in women exposed to only a few rads of radiation.[23] For perspective, it should be noted that routine chest x-rays and, with new techniques, mammography have radiation exposures under 1 rad.

Most observers believe that it is unlikely that radiation exposure is responsible for any appreciable proportion of the cases of breast cancer in the general population.[24] In view of the data, as a general recommendation, radiation to the breast, especially in young females, should be avoided.[25] This should not be construed to imply that mammography should be avoided. As will be discussed, mammography utilizes low-dose radiation and is a recommended screening technique for the detection of early breast cancer in specific situations.

ORAL CONTRACEPTIVES AND BREAST CANCER

Because of the suspected link between hormones and breast cancer, there have been numerous studies undertaken to evaluate the possible relationship between oral contraceptives (which generally are combinations of two hormones) and breast cancer. Nineteen experts on the epidemiology of breast cancer, who together form the "Multidisciplinary Project on Breast Cancer of the International Union against Cancer," met recently and reviewed the data.[26] They reported that studies show no overall increase in risk associated with the use of oral contraceptives. There have been some reports of an increased risk in several specific categories of women, for example, women with benign breast disease. The committee points out that after detailed analysis even these results are not consistent. They further caution that findings from previous studies may have little present relevance because of the substantial changes in the formulation of birth control pills over the years. In particular, the doses of hormones are much lower today than in earlier versions of "the pill." Thus, the panel's report states, "It may be concluded from the data now available that concern over breast cancer is not a reason for restriction of the use of oral contraceptives."

In another recent review of this problem, the author agrees that the aggregate of available information does not show any increased risk for breast cancer with the use of oral contraceptives. He also suggests that there may be some basis for believing that oral contraceptives may actually lower breast cancer risk.[27]

Available data thus far indicate that birth control pills are not a risk factor in the development of breast cancer.

FAMILY HISTORY AND BREAST CANCER

The extent to which heredity influences the development of breast cancer is an important issue. A relationship between family history and this disease has been suspected for a long time. In a review, the author relates that in 1866 Paul Broca observed that in his own family 24 women died of breast cancer.[28]

There have been many studies designed to elucidate the relationship between genetics and breast cancer. A recent Danish study of twins revealed that genetic factors were important in the development of cancer of the breast.[29] A study from Harvard compared 1159 women with breast cancer to 11,590 controls. They concluded that "having a mother with breast cancer increased a woman's risk of developing the disease by 80%, while having a sister with such a history increased the risk by 150%."[30] An increased risk for breast cancer in women with a mother or sister who had the disease was also found in a Swedish study.[31]

In their published report, a group of experts reviewed the data available on family history and breast cancer.[32] They noted that a two- to threefold increase in risk with a family history of breast cancer in first-degree relatives (mother, sister, or daughter) is widely acknowledged. Furthermore, the risk increases still further if two first-degree relatives have the disease.

It is apparent from available information that a family history of breast cancer is a risk factor in the development of this tumor. Women with a mother or sister with breast cancer should be aware that they are at increased risk. Appropriate screening measures such as breast self-examination, frequent medical examinations, and mammography should be obtained by women who know they are at high risk.

BENIGN BREAST DISEASE AND BREAST CANCER

In the past, there was some confusion about the relationship between benign breast disease and breast cancer. A study of 1441 patients with benign breast disease followed for an average of 12.9 years showed that these patients had more than twice the risk of developing breast cancer than the general population.[33]

A review of the available information by epidemiology experts showed that a two- to threefold increase in risk in women with a history of benign breast disease was a consistent finding.[34]

Women with a history of benign breast disease are at an increased risk. It is important that individuals at higher risk make use of screening examinations and practice breast self-examination.

AGE AND HEIGHT AND BREAST CANCER

The association between increasing age and a rising incidence of breast cancer has been demonstrated. In a review on the subject, it was recently noted that the risk of developing breast cancer increases with every year of life.[35]

The association of height and the risk of developing breast cancer is still disputed. Nutritional factors confound the picture somewhat since height has been clearly shown to be related to food intake. In the Netherlands, height has been consistently associated with an increased risk of developing breast cancer. However, this correlation has not been consistently demonstrated elsewhere.[36] Others disagree and feel that height is an identified and independent risk factor.[37] Overall, then, it is difficult to make a definitive statement in this area.

CONSTITUTIONAL FACTORS AND BREAST CANCER

The term *constitutional factors* is used to encompass all hormonal events in a woman's life that have been shown to be associated with either an increased risk of the development of breast cancer or to play a protective role. These include age at menarche (the beginning of menstruation), age at menopause (the cessation of menstruation), and age at the birth of the first child. The age at menarche is also mediated by nutritional factors. Improvements in nutrition correlate with a younger age at menarche.

Early menarche, late menopause, and giving birth to the first child after the age of 30 are associated with an increased risk of breast cancer. Also, the younger a woman is when she gives birth to her first child, the lower is her risk of developing breast cancer.[38,39]

All these events are known to involve hormonal changes, and breast tissue is extremely sensitive to hormonal stimulation. It is not clear what the exact mechanism is that explains the changes in risk with these events. There are many different theories.

According to one estimate, a population that achieved a 5-year reduction in average age at first delivery might experience a 30 percent reduction in the incidence of breast cancer.[40] Women who plan to have children should be informed of the advisability of having their first child by the age of *30*.

NURSING AND BREAST CANCER

It was previously thought that breast feeding played a protective role against the development of breast cancer. This is no longer believed correct. Careful modern studies show that there is no significant difference in risk between nursing mothers and those who do not nurse.[41]

An evaluation of extensive data on nursing and breast cancer obtained from an additional large case-control study also recently demonstrated the lack of a protective effect for nursing.[42]

ESTROGENS AND BREAST CANCER

The relationship between the use of "exogenous" estrogens — estrogens used as medications — and the development of breast cancer has been studied for years. Estrogens are sometimes used to decrease severity of the' symptoms of women in the premenopausal and menopausal period. They have also been used as so-called replacement estrogens after a hysterectomy that included removal of the ovaries.

Most early studies show no increased risk of breast cancer with the use of estrogens. However, recent studies show just the opposite. There is now evidence that after a latent period there is a disturbing association of estrogen use and breast cancer. One report shows a more than threefold increase in breast cancer risk in women who use estrogens.[43] Another recently published review warns of the same risk of estrogen use.[44] The report of an international group of experts concludes, "Thus there is cause for concern that the use of non-contraceptive estrogens increases the incidence of breast cancer."[45]

It has become recently apparent that estrogen usage is a risk factor in the development of breast cancer. Women currently taking these hormones should be aware of the potential danger involved. In general, it would be wise to avoid these agents. There are certain special situations in which your physician may feel the risk of using estrogens is outweighed by the potential benefit that may accrue. The weakening of bones, known as osteoporosis, which is seen in the elderly, can sometimes be helped by these agents.

RESERPINE AND BREAST CANCER

Reserpine is a drug that is sometimes used in the treatment of high blood pressure. It is one of the constituents of a commonly used combination of antihypertensive medications. There have been reports in the past suggesting a possible link between reserpine use and the development of breast cancer.

The Mayo Clinic recently extensively studied this question. Analyzing data on 2000 women with high blood pressure, they found no association between reserpine use and breast cancer. In addition, they question the validity of the previous studies that claimed such a link.[46]

It now seems conclusive that there is no link between reserpine and increased breast cancer risk.

THYROID SUPPLEMENTS AND
BREAST CANCER

Various theories have been advanced in an attempt to explain the role of homones in the development of breast cancer. In the past, there has been the suggestion that thyroid hormone might be somehow implicated. Therefore, the question of the use of thyroid medication and the risk of breast cancer was raised. Indeed, a study in 1976 reported such a link.[47]

In order to evaluate the possible association of thyroid supplements and breast cancer risk, a large case-control study was undertaken. The study compared 659 women with breast cancer and 1719 contols. The recently published analysis reveals no association between the use of thyroid supplements, even for periods greater than 15 years, and breast cancer. The investigators concluded that available data did not justify any suspicion of a link between thyroid supplements and breast cancer.[48]

There is a great body of knowledge concerning the risk factors associated with breast cancer. Risk factors in this disease are especially important since they offer the potential for modification and,

TABLE 5-4. RISK FACTORS IN THE DEVELOPMENT OF BREAST CANCER

Age

Obesity

High dietary fat intake

Late age at birth of first child (more than 30 years old)

History of benign breast disease

Estrogen use

Family history of breast cancer

Never having borne children

Early menarche (onset of menstruation)

Late menopause (cessation of menstruation)

Radiation exposure

ultimately, prevention. We have reviewed both known risk factors (Table 5-4) and suspected risk factors (Table 5-5). In the next section, we will see some practical application of this information.

TABLE 5-5. POSSIBLE RISK FACTORS IN THE DEVELOPMENT OF BREAST CANCER

Height

Exposure to a cancer-causing virus (unlikely)

WHAT YOU CAN DO

Breast cancer is a significant cause of early death and is the most common cancer North American women face. Advances in treatment have yielded little in the way of improved survival. Therefore, it is apparent that a more active role in the prevention and early diagnosis of this disease is essential.

You hold the key. There are two important ways to lessen your risk: (1) early detection and (2) active modification of risk factors.

Early Detection

Early detection of breast cancer increases the chances for cure and increased survival.[49] Most breast cancers are found by the patient herself either by accident or during breast self-examination. In contrast, the first discovery of a breast mass is much less often noted during a routine visit to your doctor.

It is extremely important that all women practice breast self-examination (Table 5-2). It has been estimated that breast cancer mortality might be reduced by 18.8 percent if all women routinely did.[50] You can readily make this a routine habit. If you have daughters, teach them the technique and its importance.

Women who are at higher risk and those more than 50 years of age should have annual mammography done. This is a low-dose x-ray of your breast that can reveal tumors before they can be felt. Based on available data, there is little danger from radiation exposure with newer mammography techniques.

Supplement both breast self-examination and mammography with frequent examinations by your physician. When you take these steps, you can go a long way toward improving your chances with breast cancer.

Active Modification of Risk Factors

The importance of nutritional factors in the development of breast cancer has become apparent. Total dietary fat intake and being overweight are particularly dangerous. Remember, you hold the key. Several authors have rightly called for an "attack on life-style" to attempt prevention of the disease.[51,52] The essential components of this step are:

1. Avoid overeating.
2. Maintain ideal weight at all ages.
3. Avoid excess consumption of fat.

This program also applies to your daughters, especially during adolescence and early adulthood.

Women who plan to have children can achieve a marked reduction in breast cancer risk by not delaying the birth of their first child.

Avoid unnecessary radiation exposure to your breasts. This is particularly important in adolescents and young women.

Estrogens should only be used in very specific situations that are determined by your doctor.

This comprehensive appoach can result in a substantial reduction in the dangers you face from breast cancer. It takes commitment but it can save your life (Table 5-6).

NEW FRONTIERS

Although breast cancer is currently a devastating disease, there are reasons to be hopeful. Advances in the treatment of breast cancer and in its earlier diagnosis augur well for improved survival. The use of systematic chemotherapeutic agents (cancer drugs) following surgery in an attempt to prolong survival and increase cure rates is promising. More aggressive chemotherapy in this setting may prove advantageous. Mass screening techniques with mammography in women over 50 or in those at high risk may detect breast cancer at an earlier stage.

Advances in information on risk factors and the utilization of this

TABLE 5-6. WHAT YOU CAN DO TO LESSEN
YOUR RISK FROM BREAST CANCER

Breast self-examination.

Mammography (if you are more than 50 or at high risk).

Regular breast examinations.

Mothers, teach your daughters breast self-examination.

Avoid overeating.

Maintain ideal weight at all ages.

Avoid excess consumption of fat.

Women who plan on having children, when circumstances allow, should not delay the birth of their firstborn.

Avoid unnecessary radiation exposure to your breasts.

Do not take estrogens.

knowledge in an attempt to prevent breast cancer represent an exciting prospect. Dietary intervention that would, from available data, lessen breast cancer incidence is an important first step. Happily, the low fat, weight-reduction diet recommended is nearly identical to that which would also be used to lessen the risk of heart disease.

YOU AND YOUR DOCTOR

The relationship between you and your doctor is an important one in the successful detection of breast cancer.

Your physician can teach you breast self-examination and help guide you in a low-fat diet and weight-loss program. These are significant elements in the prevention program that has been outlined.

In the event a breast mass is detected, your doctor may need to obtain a biopsy. A biopsy is the surgical removal of the involved breast tissue for examination under a microscope. This examination will reveal if the mass is benign or malignant. Most breast masses are benign.

If breast cancer is present, surgery may be recommended. There are several types of surgical procedures in current use (Table 5-7). Remember, you can take an active role in lessening the risk of your developing breast cancer. Use the information contained in this chapter to protect yourself and your daughters.

TABLE 5-7. THE TYPES OF MASTECTOMY

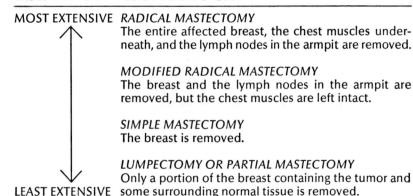

MOST EXTENSIVE *RADICAL MASTECTOMY*
The entire affected breast, the chest muscles underneath, and the lymph nodes in the armpit are removed.

MODIFIED RADICAL MASTECTOMY
The breast and the lymph nodes in the armpit are removed, but the chest muscles are left intact.

SIMPLE MASTECTOMY
The breast is removed.

LUMPECTOMY OR PARTIAL MASTECTOMY
Only a portion of the breast containing the tumor and
LEAST EXTENSIVE some surrounding normal tissue is removed.

REFERENCES

1. Yonemoto R: Breast cancer in Japan and the United States. *Archieves of Surgery* 115: 1056–1061, 1980.
2. Miller AB: Breast cancer, *Cancer* 47:1109–1113, 1981.
3. Wynder E: Dietary factors related to breast cancer. *Cancer* 46:899–904, 1980.
4. Cole P: Major aspects of the epidemiology of breast cancer. *Cancer* 46:865–867, 1980.
5. Nasca P, et al: Relationship of hair dye use, benign breast disease, and breast cancer. *Journal of the National Cancer Institute* 64: 23–28, 1980.
6. Hennekens C, et al: Use of permanent hair dyes and cancer among registered nurses. *Lancet* July 30, 1979; 1390.
7. Stavraky K, et al: Case-controlled study of hair dye use by patients with breast cancer and endometrial cancer. *Journal of the National Cancer Institute* 63:941–945, 1979.
8. Nasca P, et al: Relationship of hair dye use, benign breast disease, and breast cancer. *Journal of the National Cancer Institute* 64:23–28, 1980.

9. Cole P: Major aspects of the epidemiology of breast cancer. *Cancer* 46:865–867, 1980.

10. Miller A, et al: Special report: the epidemiology and etiology of breast cancer. *New England Journal of Medicine* 303:1246–1248, 1980.

11. Gompel C: Epidemiology and biology of breast cancer. *Acta Chirugica Belgica* 79: 73–76, 1980.

12. Garofalo J, et al: Serum, zinc, copper, and the Cu/Zu ratio in patients with benign and malignant breast lesions. *Cancer* 46:2682–2685, 1980.

13. Garofalo J, et al: Serum, zinc, copper, and the Cu/Zu ratio in patients with benign and malignant breast lesions. *Cancer* 46:2682–2685, 1980.

14. Tartter P, et al: Cholesterol and obesity as prognostic factors in breast cancer. *Cancer* 47:2222–2227, 1981.

15. Gray CE, et al: Breast-cancer incidence and mortality rates in different countries in relation to known risk factors and dietary practices. *British Journal of Cancer* 39:1–7, 1979.

16. Yonemoto R: Breast cancer in Japan and the United States. *Archives of Surgery* 115:1056–1061, 1980.

17. Yonemoto R: Breast cancer in Japan and the United States. *Archives of Surgery* 115:1056–1061, 1980.

18. Wynder E: Dietary factors related to breast cancer. *Cancer* 46:899–904, 1980.

19. Tartter P, et al: Cholesterol and obesity as prognostic factors in breast cancer. *Cancer* 47:2222–2227, 1981.

20. Miller A, et al: Special report: the epidemiology and etiology of breast cancer. *New England Journal of Medicine* 303:1246–1248, 1980.

21. Land C: Low-dose radiation—a cause of breast cancer? *Cancer* 46:868–873, 1980.

22. Mammography Screening for Breast Cancer. *The Medical Letter*, June 27, 1980: 53–54.

23. Land, C.: Low-dose radiation—a cause of breast cancer? *Cancer* 46:868–873, 1980.

24. Cole P: Major aspects of the epidemiology of breast cancer. *Cancer* 46:865–867, 1980.

25. Miller A, et al: Special report: the epidemiology and etiology of breast cancer. *New England Journal of Medicine* 303:1246–1248, 1980.

26. Miller A, et al: Special report: the epidemiology and etiology of breast cancer. *New England Journal of Medicine* 303:1246–1248, 1980.

27. Cole P: Major aspects of the epidemiology of breast cancer. *Cancer* 46:865–867, 1980.

28. Gompel C: Epidemiology and biology of breast cancer. *Acta Chirurgica Belgica* 79:73–76, 1980.

29. Holm N, et al: Etiologic factors of breast cancer elucidated by a study of

unselected twins. *Journal of the National Cancer Institute* 65:285–298, 1980.

30. Bain C, et al: Family history of breast cancer as a risk indicator for the disease. *American Journal of Epidemiology* 111: 1980.

31. Adam HO, et al: Familiality in breast cancer: a case-control study in a Swedish population. *British Journal of Cancer* 42: 1980.

32. Miller A, et al: Special report: the epidemiology and etiology of breast cancer. *New England Journal of Medicine* 303:1246–1248, 1980.

33. Hutchinson W, et al: Risk of breast cancer in women with benign breast disease. *Journal of the National Cancer Institute* 65: 13–20, 1980.

34. Miller A, et al: Special report: the epidemiology and etiology of breast cancer. *New England Journal of Medicine* 303:1246–1248, 1980.

35. Gompel C: Epidemiology and biology of breast cancer. *Acta Chirugica Belgica* 79:73–76, 1980.

36. Miller A, et al: Special report: the epidemiology and etiology of breast cancer. *New England Journal of Medicine* 303:1246–1248, 1980.

37. Tartter P, et al: Cholesterol and obesity as prognostic factors in breast cancer. *Cancer* 47:2222–2227, 1981.

38. Miller A, et al: Special report: the epidemiology and etiology of breast cancer. *New England Journal of Medicine* 303:1246–1248, 1980.

39. Cole P: Major aspects of the epidemiology of breast cancer. *Cancer* 46:865–867, 1980.

40. Miller A, et al: Special report: the epidemiology and etiology of breast cancer. *New England Journal of Medicine* 303:1246–1248, 1980.

41. Gompel C: Epidemiology and biology of breast cancer. *Acta Chirugica Belgica* 79:73–76, 1980.

42. Kalache A, et al: Short reports: reason for variable response to tine test, *British Medical Journal* January 26, 1980; 223–224.

43. Hershel J, et al: Replacement estrogens and breast cancer. *American Journal of Epidemiology* 112:586–594, 1980.

44. Cole P: Major aspects of the epidemiology of breast cancer. *Cancer* 46:865–867, 1980.

45. Miller A, et al: Special report: the epidemiology and etiology of breast cancer. *New England Journal of Medicine* 303:1246–1248, 1980.

46. Labarthe D, et al: Reserpine and breast cancer. *JAMA* 243:2304–2310, 1980.

47. Kapd CC, et al: Breast cancer: relationship to thyroid supplements for hypothyroidism. *JAMA* 236:1124–1127, 1976.

48. Shapiro S, et al: Use of thyroid supplements in relation to the risk of breast cancer. *JAMA* 224:1685–1687, 1980.

49. Nasca P: Current status of breast cancer screening. *Current Concepts in Oncology* March/April 1981:17–19.

50. Nasca P: Current status of breast cancer screening. *Current Concepts in Oncology* March/April 1981:17–19.

51. Miller A: Breast cancer. *Cancer* 47:1109–1113, 1981.

52. Miller A, et al: Special report: the epidemiology and etiology of breast cancer. *New England Journal of Medicine* 303:1246–1248, 1980.

53. Kirkland, DJ, et al: *Lancet* 11:124, 1978.

54. National Cancer Institute, *Carcinogenesis Testing Program.* Washington, DC, US Government Printing Office, 1978.

SIX

Lung Cancer

At the turn of the century, lung cancer was so rare that in a monograph reviewing the disease only 374 cases could be collected from the world's literature; the author apologized for writing about such an uncommon disease. The writer, Adler, was the first person in 1912 to associate these tumors with smoking cigarettes. Today, lung cancer is the leading cause of cancer deaths among U.S. men. In this decade, lung cancer will exceed breast cancer as the major cause of death from cancer in women as well.[1] Between 1945 and 1975, the U.S. lung cancer death rates exploded fivefold, creating a situation that the U.S. Public Health Service has called "an alarming epidemic." More than 100,000 men and women will be stricken with lung cancer this year.[2] It is the most common deadly tumor in an increasing number of countries.

Most of these people will die of their disease. The median survival from time of diagnosis remains under 6 months, and at 5 years from diagnosis, barely 10 percent of patients are still alive. Yet this scourge of death need not happen. Lung cancer is largely preventable, with more than 80 percent of cases attributable to cigarette smoking. There is absolutely no doubt about the clear-cut and deadly relationship between smoking and lung cancer. In the 1979 U.S. Surgeon General's Report on smoking, it is again confirmed that the death rate of U.S. men who smoke cigarettes is ten times higher for lung cancer.[1]

The more cigarettes you smoke, the greater is your danger of developing cancer of the lung. Hammond and Horn reported that the death rate from cancer of the lung per hundred thousand is 3.4 in the male nonsmoker, 59.3 for 10 to 20 cigarettes per day, and 217.3 for 40 or more cigarettes per day.[3] This demonstrates the so-called dose-response relationship between cigarette smoking and lung cancer. In other words, the more one smokes as measured by total pack years of smoking, number of cigarettes per day, the amount inhaled, and the age at starting smoking, the greater the risk (Table 6-1).

It has also been repeatedly demonstrated that if you stop smoking, you are less likely to develop lung cancer than someone who continues to smoke. The risk of lung cancer decreases after the cessation of smoking, almost to the level of the nonsmoker; the time this takes depends on the amount and years of smoking prior to stopping. This decreased risk is seen even with very heavy smokers. In Great Britain, a survey of 600,000 physicians revealed that between 1951 and 1965 approximately one-half gave up smoking. Overall death rates for tobacco-associated disease fell markedly in this group. The lung cancer

TABLE 6-1. SMOKING CHARACTERISTICS THAT INCREASE THE RISK OF A CIGARETTE SMOKER'S DEVELOPING CANCER OF THE LUNG

The number of cigarettes smoked

Early age of beginning the smoking habit

Number of years smoking

The amount of smoke inhaled

Individual smoking peculiarities (the particular "style" of smoking. For example, in England, where smokers smoke a cigarette to the butt, there is a much greater incidence of lung cancer.)

All of these factors can increase the risk of developing lung cancer to the individual smoker. They are really measures of the "amount" smoked. This illustrates the "dose-response" relationship between the "dose" of tobacco smoke and the development of lung cancer.

mortality rate among these physicians plunged 38 percent, while at the same time the death rate from lung cancer for all men in England and Wales who had not changed their smoking habits climbed 7 percent.[4]

The cellular changes leading to lung cancer are apparently progressive and reversible. In other words, there is a slow process of continued injury to cells in the lung. This results in damage and increasing cellular response. At some point, there is conversion of normal cells to cancer cells. It is at this point and only at this point that the damage is irreversible. However, prior to this malignant change, simply stopping smoking will result in the reversal of the process (Table 6-2). The risk of lung cancer even for people who have smoked as long as 30 to 40 years declines after 10 years of not smoking, while in those who smoke less, the risk declines as early as 1 to 4 years after stopping the habit.[4]

TABLE 6-2. CELLULAR CHANGES IN THE LUNG LEADING TO CANCER

Normal

Nonspecific inflammatory reaction

Nonspecific reactive hyperplasia and metaplasia (increase in cells with some changes but no cancer or malignant changes)

Increasing atypia (abnormal cells; these changes are present in 93 percent of active smokers, 6 percent of ex-smokers 5 to 15 years after they stopped smoking and 1 percent of nonsmokers)

Localized cancer (carcinoma in situ)

Invasive cancer (invasive carcinoma)

Note that the changes leading to cancer were present in 93 percent of active smokers but only 6 percent of ex-smokers and 1 percent of nonsmokers. In other words, prior to the development of cancer, if you stop smoking the changes are reversible.

Adapted from Holland.[5]

Although cigarette smoking is clearly the major cause of lung cancer, attention has been directed to other factors such as air pollution, radiation, and cancer-causing agents in the environment and workplace. Some environmental agents have been associated with the development of lung cancer (Table 6-3). There has been no demonstrable association between lung cancer and air pollution.[4]

TABLE 6-3. ENVIRONMENTAL AGENTS ASSOCIATED WITH LUNG CANCER (RISK FACTORS)

Cigarette smoking

Pipe and tobacco smoking

Asbestos (mining, pipe fitting, shipyards)

Uranium (mining of uranium ore)

Nickel (ore and refining)

Tar and coal fumes

Zinc exposure (common air contaminant, industrial uses)

Iron oxides (factory workers, metal grinders)

Chromium compounds (ore, glass workers)

Beryllium (fluorescent powders, lamps and sign tubes, casting beryllium alloys, and extraction of beryllium from its ore)

Bis (chloromethyl) ether

A greatly increased risk of lung cancer is faced by an individual who is exposed to these materials and is a smoker. This has been clearly demonstrated among asbestos workers and uranium miners.

Adapted from Holland,[5] Schottenfeld,[4] and Wintrobe.[3]

WHAT IS LUNG CANCER?

Lung cancer was the apparent underlying cause of an illness that struck miners in Schneeburg Saxony as early as 1420.[5] This malady was seen in the miners after working in the mines for approximately 20 years; they became short of breath and had to change jobs. In 1879, the disease's true nature was recognized and termed "sarcoma" and later carcinoma. Physicians in the nineteenth century generally recognized the existence of lung cancer as a rare and untreatable disease.

Your lungs play a vital role in maintaining life. They serve to exchange carbon dioxide, a cellular waste product, with oxygen, needed for the maintenance of metabolic cellular activity. Inhaled air containing oxygen enters the body through the nose and mouth. From there, the air travels down various breathing tubes until reaching the small air sacs known as alveoli where the exchange between oxygen and carbon dioxide takes place. The main air passageway, known as the trachea, divides into the right and left bronchus to supply the right and left lung, respectively.

Normally, the cells lining these passages as well as other cells in the body grow in an orderly, controlled pattern. The controlled growth and reproduction are a necessary cycle that allows new cells to replace old and worn-out cells. In lung cancer, as in other cancer, there is an uncontrolled growth and reproduction of abnormal cells. These cells are not limited by boundaries that inhibit normal cells. Thus, they are capable of "invading" normal cells and of spreading throughout the body. The process of tumor cells spreading is termed metastasis.

Cancer of the lung can spread in any of four ways:

1. Direct growth and extension into neighboring (contiguous) tissues
2. Through the blood (hematogenous)
3. Through the lymph system (lymphatic)
4. Rarely through the air passages (transbronchial)

Different cancers have preferential sites of spread. In lung cancer, favorite sites include the brain, liver, bones, adrenal glands, and lymph glands (Table 6-4).

There are different types of lung cancer. The particular types are classified according to their appearance under the microscope. They each have particular characteristics in their clinical behavior (the way they manifest themselves and spread within the body) as well. There are some variations among authorities about classification. However,

TABLE 6-4. COMMON SITES OF TUMOR SPREAD IN LUNG CANCER

Brain

Liver

Adrenal glands

Prescalene lymph nodes (lymph glands in the area of the first rib in front)
Bone

Symptoms vary according to the site of spread. For example, in spread to the brain, there may be convulsions, headache, nausea, personality changes, blurred vision, double vision, and paralysis. Whereas in spread to the bone, there may be only bone pain.

the concept is useful in describing, predicting, and treating different types of cancer of the lung. The clinical presentation of lung cancer depends to a large extent on cell type. We have divided cancer of the lung into four major types (Table 6-5):

1. Squamous cell
2. Undifferentiated or anaplastic
3. Adenocarcinoma
4. Bronchoalveolar (alveolar cell; relatively rare).

All these types are associated with cigarette smoking; however, types 1 and 2 have the strongest link.

TABLE 6-5. MAJOR CELL TYPES OF LUNG CANCER

Squamous (or epidermoid)—this type has the slowest growth rate and the lowest incidence of distant spread by blood. It usually occurs in a central position and because of this produces earlier symptoms. Spread is generally by continuity, and the lesion may cavitate. It is strongly associated with cigarette smoking and represents 35 to 60 percent of all lung cancer.

Undifferentiated or anaplastic (includes round cell or large cell and oat cell [small cell] type—this type has rapid growth with very early distant spread by both blood and lymph vessels. It is responsive to radiation therapy and combination chemotherapy. The tumor occurs equally in central and peripheral locations in the lung field. At the time of diagnosis, distant spread is present in more than 90 percent of the tumors of the oat cell variety. It represents 20 to 30 percent of all lung cancer.

Adenocarcinoma—this tumor occurs usually in peripheral locations in the lung field. It has been associated with focal lung scans and fibrosis "scar carcinoma." This type may spread by all routes but particularly by the blood stream and often remains clinically silent until distant hematogenous (blood borne) spread occurs. Adenocarcinoma represents 15 to 20 percent of all lung cancer.

Bronchioalveolar cell—this type is uncommon and represents only 2 percent of all lung cancer. It is usually diffuse or multinodular. There is significant shortness of breath and rapid breathing associated with this tumor.

The classification of cell types of lung cancer varies considerably. Many divide the undifferentiated into its component oat cell and large cell types. The relative percentage of each type, as noted in the literature, also varies somewhat from study to study.

SIGNS AND SYMPTOMS OF LUNG CANCER

Early diagnosis is extremely important in any attempt to improve the abysmal cure rate for lung cancer. It is very important for you to be aware of the signs and symptoms of lung cancer. Awareness could bring earlier detection; earlier detection increases your chances of successful treatment.

The constellation of symptoms and signs that result from lung cancer is, as we've mentioned, dependent on many factors, including cell type, location within the lung, and the "biologic predetermination" of the tumor itself. These symptom complexes can be divided into "early" and "late" presentations.[3] It should be remembered that lung cancer often develops with few signs and symptoms, so that the diagnosis is only suspected on the basis of a chest x-ray obtained during a routine checkup.

The "early" presentation of lung cancer is of particular importance. Awareness of early symptoms offers the most potential for successful treatment. At this point in the disease, many of the signs and symptoms are subtle. Partial obstruction inside a small airway, for example, could lead to a change in the pattern of an already-present cigarette cough. The problem is that many symptoms like cough, chest

TABLE 6-6. SYMPTOMS OF "EARLY" LUNG CANCER

Mild cough

Change in pattern of a cigarette cough

Persistent chest pain or ache

Fever

Chills

Sputum production

Localized wheeze (noise accompanying breathing)

Coughing up blood-tinged sputum (hemoptysis)

Recurring attacks of pneumonia or bronchitis

In many patients, there are no early symptoms, and the physician examination may be normal. The diagnosis is often suspected on the basis of an abnormal chest x-ray during a routine checkup.

Adapted from Wintrobe.[3]

pain, and sputum production are accepted as normal to the long-time smoker (who is exactly the person at risk). The development of symptoms also depends on the location within the lung field in which the tumor develops. Central lesions produce earlier symptoms because of obstruction to the larger airways (Table 6-6).

The "late" presentation of lung cancer is ominous in that the tumor has, at this stage, frequently spread beyond the point at which curative surgery is possible. The clinical presentation depends on the cell type and tumor size and spread (metastasis; Table 6-4). There are four ways in which the tumor can manifest itself:

1. Nonspecific systemic symptoms
2. Signs and symptoms of spread within the chest
3. Signs and symptoms of spread beyond the chest (eg, bone, brain, liver, adrenals, etc)
4. The very interesting "classical" systemic syndrome (Table 6-7).

A person with advanced lung cancer can manifest his disease with a variety of nonspecific symptoms. These symptoms include weight

TABLE 6-7. SYMPTOMS OF "LATE" LUNG CANCER

Weight loss

Loss of appetite (anorexia)

Nausea and vomiting

Weakness and fatigue

Hoarseness

Pleurisy (pleuritis)

Difficulty swallowing (dysphagia)

Syndrome characterized by drooping eyelid, decreased sweating on the affected side of the face, contracted pupil, and recession of the eyeball within the socket (Horner's syndrome)

Collapsed lung (atelectasis)

Systemic syndromes (Table 6-8)

Systems of tumor spread (metastases: these symptoms depend on the sites and extent of spread—Table 6-4)

loss, loss of appetite, nausea, vomiting, and weakness. The longer these symptoms persist, the less likely it is that the tumor can be surgically removed.

When the tumor has spread within the chest cavity, there is another group of symptoms that may appear. In this situation, the person may be hoarse for a sustained period, have a paralyzed diaphragm on one side, have difficulty swallowing, or have fluid in the lung or pleurisy. Sometimes Horner's syndrome is seen when nerves from the neck region of the spinal cord are involved. In this syndrome, there is a strange combination of signs, including drooping eyelid, decreased sweating of the face on the affected side, contracted pupil,

TABLE 6-8. SYSTEMIC SYNDROMES ASSOCIATED WITH CANCER OF THE LUNG

High blood calcium (hypercalcemia)

Low blood sodium in combination with a high urine concentration (inappropriate ADH)

Syndrome of abnormal sugar metabolism, purple skin striations, obesity of the trunk and face with "buffalo hump" distribution, high blood pressure and "thinning" of the bones (Cushing's syndrome)

Enlarged breasts (gynecomastia)

Syndrome of wheezing, diarrhea, and flushing (carcinoid syndrome seen with bronchial adenoma)

Blood and blood vessel abnormalities (thrombocytopenic purpura, leukemoid reaction, myelophthisic anemia, nonbacterial thrombotic endocarditis)

Muscle weakness (peripheral neuropathy, corticocerebellar dengeration, nonspecific myopathy)

Clubbing of the fingers and toes (hypertrophic pulmonary osteoarthropathy)

Joint pain (arthralgias)

Skin abnormalities (dermatomyositis, acanthosis nigricans)

Swelling of the face, neck, and upper arms due to obstruction of the major vein draining the upper part of the body (superior vena cava obstruction)

Many of these syndromes disappear with surgical removal of the tumor or effective therapy by drugs or radiation. They often recur either locally or by distant spread (metastasis) when the tumor returns.

Adapted from Wintrobe.[3]

and sunken eyeball. Occasionally, the tumor obstructs the major vein draining the upper portion of the body. In this situation, the face, neck, upper arms, and body become swollen. (This is known as superior vena cava obstruction.)

Symptoms of spread beyond the chest are variable and depend on the site of spread (metastasis, Table 6-4). As noted previously, the most common sites of spread in cancer of the lung include the brain, liver, bones, lymph glands, and adrenal glands.

Perhaps the most interesting manifestations of advanced lung cancer are the numerous systemic syndromes (Table 6-8). Fascinating in their various manifestations, they are of clinical importance as well. Occasionally, these syndromes can appear prior to the development of a mass on chest x-ray. These syndromes often remit with effective therapy and recur when the tumor progresses. Let's take a look at some of them.[5]

Hypercalcemia or High Blood Calcium
Elevated levels of calcium in the blood are seen in 5 to 10 percent of lung cancer patients and almost always with the squamous (or epidermoid) cell type. People with elevated calcium may lose their appetite, become nauseous , be sleepy, be constipated, urinate a lot, and drink a lot. The high levels of calcium are not related to tumor in the bones despite intensive searches for this. It appears that the tumor in these cases is capable of manufacturing a hormonelike substance that raises the blood calcium levels.

Cushing's Syndrome or
Ectopic (Inappropriate) ACTH Syndrome
The relationship between this syndrome and lung cancer was first described in 1928. Most of these cases are associated with the oat-cell type of lung cancer (a type of undifferentiated or anaplastic tumor). Cushing's syndrome is a clinical manifestation of the overproduction of the hormones produced by the outer portion (cortex) of the adrenal glands. Features of this syndrome include skin striae, pigmentation, obesity, washed-out bones (osteoporosis), low blood potassium, impaired metabolism of sugar (similar to that seen in sugar diabetes), and high blood pressure. The particular signs that appear in any given person are variable. These signs, as in most of the other syndromes, disappear or lessen with successful treatment of the tumor.

Ectopic ADH Syndrome

This syndrome is also most often seen in the oat cell type of lung cancer. The tumor in these cases synthesizes a substance that acts like "antidiuretic hormone" (ADH), which interferes with the ability of the kidney to excrete water. The result is a combination of low blood sodium and increased urine concentration. These biochemical abnormalities can manifest themselves as loss of appetite, nausea, and vomiting and lethargy.

Clubbing of the Fingers and Toes, or Pulmonary Hypertrophic Osteoarthropathy

This can occur in all cell types but rarely in the oat-cell variety. Five to 12 percent of lung cancer patients will manifest these changes. Pain in the bones or joints is common and may be severe. Rapid pain relief accompanies the successful treatment of the tumor.

There are many other system syndromes (Table 6-8) that may be present. We have touched on a few interesting ones to show the protean nature of manifestations that lung cancer can have. Lung cancer is unique in this respect and also in the paradoxical situation in which it is an almost universally deadly disease that is almost completely preventable.

RISK FACTORS IN LUNG CANCER

You have already seen the dramatic association between cigarette smoking and lung cancer. But what about other risk factors linked to the development of lung cancer?

In the very beginning of this chapter, we talked about the Saxony miners who developed lung cancer. The cause of that cancer was the subject of controversy for a great many years. Variously blamed were cobalt, nickel, arsenic, and the fungus *Aspergillus*. The Saxony mines were the source of many riches, including silver; they were also the source of uranium for the experiments of Eve Curie. It was later noted that uranium miners in other areas also had a higher incidence of lung cancer. In this way, uranium was found to be a cancer-causing (carcinogenic) element in the work environment. Although the risk of lung cancer is increased in uranium miners, it is tremendously increased in uranium miners who smoke. Uranium miners who smoke face a tenfold greater risk compared to nonsmoking uranium miners (who are already at high risk). Lung cancer has been associated with many other environmental factors (Table 6-3). In all these situations, smokers who are exposed to those agents are at a markedly increased risk. If you are or *have been* exposed to any of these materials, *stop smoking.* Your risk is dramatically increased if you don't.

Asbestos is a particularly dangerous environmental carcinogen. It can cause the development of tumors 20 to 30 years after exposure and is found in many products and occupations.[6,7] Let's take a closer look.[8,9]

Asbestos is the name given a group of minerals found together as masses of almost indestructible, heat-proof, and fireproof fibers. These fibers can break into tiny particles of dust, a carcinogenic dust. The dust can float in the air, stick to clothes, and be inhaled or swallowed.

Because of its properties, asbestos has been widely used in many industries during the past 40 years. It has been utilized as insulation and for fireproofing in textiles and constructions and in the shipbuilding industry where it is used for insulating boilers, steampipes, hot-water pipes and nuclear reactors in ships. It has found its way into 300 diverse products, from potholders and children's toys to welding rods (Table 6-9).

Workers in shipyards, asbestos manufacturing, and the asbestos textile industry have shown a greater incidence of lung cancer. Smokers who have been exposed to asbestos face a fivefold increase in risk over the already high risk of smokers. From another perspective, asbestos workers who smoke are 30 to 90 times more likely to develop

TABLE 6-9. COMMON USES OF ASBESTOS

Coverings for pipes and surfaces (in new construction of ships, repairs, and refittings); insulation in construction, powerhouses and chemical plants, and for engines, hulls, and decks of ships; coatings for cables and electric wires; and putties, caulks, paints, and cement

Floor and ceiling tiles, sealants, pipe covering, and patching tape compounds

Friction products such as clutch facings, brake linings for automobiles, railroad cars and airplanes; filtration materials and theater curtains

A wide variety of asbestos cement materials and wall boards

Adapted from Asbestos Exposure (What It Means, What To Do), U.S. Dept. of Health, Education and Welfare, N.C.I., DHEW Publ. #(NIH) 7:1594

lung cancer than nonexposed nonsmokers. There is experimental evidence that this enormous risk to smoking workers can be reduced by as much as half if you stop smoking.[8] In other words, if you were exposed to asbestos on the job anytime in your life or if you think you were, you should stop smoking.

Asbestos that is found in finished products does not represent a health hazard unless the product is damaged so that fibers are exposed into the air.

THE TREATMENT OF LUNG CANCER

After a thorough evaluation, there are three currently accepted methods of treatment. They are the surgical removal of the tumor, treatment with drugs (chemotherapy), and treatment with high-energy rays (radiation therapy). The choice of the appropriate therapy or combination of therapies depends on the tumor cell type, the extent of spread at the time of diagnosis, and the ability of the patient to undergo the treatment.

Surgery

Surgery, if possible, is the preferred method of treatment of lung cancer, for it offers the possibility of a cure. The first successful removal of a lung for cancer took place in 1933 by Graham.[5] The patient was a doctor who returned to private practice and lived an additional 29 years. At his death, no tumor was found at autopsy. His surgeon ironically died before him of cancer of the lung.

Radiation therapy can be used in the treatment of metastases, for example, bony lesions, for the relief of pain. It can also be used in combination with surgery or chemotherapy.

Chemotherapy

Chemotherapy is simply the use of drugs to kill cancer cells. These drug treatments can be used alone or in combination with either surgery or radiation or both. The drugs also injure normal cells, so that your doctor must be skilled in balancing the harmful effects with "tumor kill." Common side effects of treatment include nausea and vomiting, diarrhea, hair loss, anemia, susceptibility to bleeding, and infections and mouth sores. Individuals tolerate chemotherapy differently, and the side effects depend on the particular drugs used and their dosages. Most side effects disappear when the drugs are stopped. For example, hair will regrow, and mouth sores will heal. If you are on chemotherapy, it is important to take any fever or elevation in temperature you have seriously; report these to your doctor immediately.

YOU AND YOUR DOCTOR

Your doctor has the task of suspecting the diagnosis and guiding you to appropriate specialists for evaluation and treatment. There are three types of specialists who may become involved in your care: the medical oncologist, who is an expert in the use of drugs and chemotherapy; the surgeon, who plays a key role in both evaluation and treatment; and the radiotherapist, who is an expert in the use of radiotherapy to kill tumor cells. Working together, these doctors can do much to offer you the best possible chances for cure or enhanced survival. There are three principal goals in the diagnostic evaluation, prior to therapy, of a patient with suspected lung cancer.[3]

1. Identification of the lesion as cancer with tissue confirmation (Before therapy, microscopic evaluation of the tumor to determine if it is cancerous and to identify the specific cell type is important.)
2. Determination of the extent of tumor spread, that is, whether the tumor has extended (a) within the lungs (so that the lung is no longer surgically resectable) and (b) beyond the chest (metastatic spread)
3. Preoperative evaluation of the patient to determine whether he can tolerate the planned removal of lung tissue

There are many tools available to your doctor to help in these goals. In most cases, the initial diagnostic approach is through various x-ray studies. There are many different types of x-rays available providing different angles and views of the lung to help visualize a tumor mass. In many cases, an abnormal chest x-ray is the only finding in a person who has no symptoms. Let's take a look at some of the studies your doctor may order in his evaluation.

Chest x-ray. This is the most widely used test and offers the best screening for lung cancer that is currently available. The chest x-ray is a regular part of a routine checkup, and in the case of heavy smokers, who are at particular risk, this study may be repeated every six months. *Tomograms.* This is a special x-ray study of the lungs that can be invaluable in the evaluation of a tumor growth. It demonstrates "slices" or layers of the lungs one at a time. In this way, it may reveal a small tumor not visible on a plain chest x-ray and give clues as to the nature of any mass present (presence of calcification, etc). When these views are taken together, they give a three-dimensional picture of the lungs and any mass within them.

Bronchoscopy

This is very helpful in the evaluation of lung cancer and along with *mediastinoscopy* and *sputum cytology* plays a key role in the evaluation of a patient. The bronchoscope is a flexible, thin tube that is passed into the smaller branches of the lung airways. The physician passing the tube has a viewer through which he can visualize the inside of these airways. This technique helps locate otherwise hidden tumors and can be used to remove a section of suspected tumor for evaluation under a microscope. The instrument allows for "brushings" and "washings" of suspected areas that free cells for microscopic evaluation.

Mediastinoscopy

This is a procedure that is used to both establish a diagnosis and evaluate the extent of spread (stage) in a patient with lung cancer. It utilizes an instrument that allows the visualization of structures between the lungs and the back of the heart. The use of this procedure before surgery has allowed for a more accurate determination of whether surgical resection of the tumor is possible. The presence of lymph glands invaded by a tumor in this area help identify a patient as having a nonresectable (inoperable) tumor and may spare a patient needless surgery.

Sputum Cytology

This is the microscopic evaluation of a patient's sputum. The sputum is examined under a microscopic to search for abnormal-appearing cells. In a fashion similar to the Papanicolaou smear for cancer of the cervix, it can offer an early clue to the presence of cancer. It is the least invasive test available for making the diagnosis of cancer. It is most useful when the tumor (1) is located in the upper portion of the lung, (2) communicates with a large airway, (3) has a large size. The combination of bronchoscopy, mediastinoscopy, and sputum cytology is estimated to provide a positive diagnosis in more than 80 percent of all patients with the squamous cell variety of lung cancer.

Thoracotomy

This is the surgical procedure in which the chest is opened for exploration and, if possible, removal of the tumor. It is a major operation but in today's times is relatively safe, having a less than 1 percent mortality rate. Frequently, patients can return home in 10 to 14 days and resume work in 6 weeks.

There are other tests your doctor may order, depending on the individual aspects of your case. Don't be afraid to ask questions. The U.S. Department of Health Education and Welfare has published a list of questions you may wish to ask your doctor.[10] They are:

- What kind of cancer do I have?
- Is the tumor benign or malignant?
- If it is benign, has it been cured?
- If it is cancer, has it spread?
- Can you predict how successful an operation or radiation treatment would be?
- What are the risks?
- Should I get an opinion from another doctor?
- If an operation is done, will I need other treatment?
- How helpful will this be in resuming normal activities afterward?
- If I take anticancer drugs, what will the side effects be?
- How often will I need medical checkups?
- What should I tell my relatives and friends?

If you or someone you love smokes: *Stop!*

Don't be a victim of expert multimillion-dollar marketing techniques. There are no crystal-clear mountain lakes or wild horses (as depicted in advertisements) on the cancer wards.

REFERENCES

1. Tobacco — hazards to health and human reproduction. *Population Reports*, Series 1, #1, 3/79.

2. Cancer facts and figures. *American Cancer Society*, 1978.

3. Wintrobe MM, et al (eds): *Principles of Internal Medicine*, ed 8, 1977.

4. Schottenfeld D, *Cancer Epidemiology and Prevention, Current Concepts.*

5. Holland J, et al: *Cancer Medicine* 1473–1518, 1973.

6. Blot W, et al: Original contributions — geographic patterns of lung cancer: industrial correlations, *American Journal of epidemiology* 103: 1976.

7. Blot W, et al: Lung cancer after employment in shipyards during World War II. *New England Journal of Medicine*, 1978.

8. Asbestos exposure, what it means, what to do, National Cancer Institute, DHEW Publ. #(NIH) 78–1594.

9. Anton TJ: *Occupational Safety and Health Management.* 1979, pp. 157–159.

SEVEN

Colon Cancer

With the exception of skin cancer, cancer of the colon (large bowel) and rectum is the most common cancer in the United States. One out of every 20 Americans will develop cancer of the colon and rectum.[1] Estimates indicate that this tumor will be diagnosed in more than 115,000 people this year and 60 percent of these will die of their disease within 5 years.[2] From another perspective, only lung cancer in men and breast cancer in women are responsible for more cancer deaths than cancer of the colon and rectum. Both men and women are equally at risk.

The tumor is recognized as having worldwide importance. The populations of Western and affluent industrial nations are at particular risk. There is a widespread international variation in the incidence of cancer of the colon and rectum. However, individuals who migrate to other countries generally assume the colon cancer risk of their adopted country.

There is a great deal of evidence to indicate that there are significant environmental factors at work in the etiology of colon cancer. It is also known that there are predisposing diseases and genetic factors that may place particular individuals at risk. Thus, this tumor has both environmental and genetic factors strongly implicated in its development. Cancer of the colon has a very poor 5-year survival rate. In addition, there does not appear to be any immediate prospect for dramatic breakthroughs in therapy. It is generally believed that the poor outcome associated with this disease is a result of the advanced stages of the tumor that are present by the time symptoms appear and medical attention is sought.

There are reasons for optimism in the exploration of two unique and unrelated approaches to this problem.

Screening and early diagnosis of cancer of the colon and rectum represent an important new approach to the treatment of this tumor. Remember that the low 5-year survival of 42 percent is thought to be largely related to late diagnosis.[3] New techniques are now available that make possible the screening of large numbers of people without symptoms. In addition, the identification of groups at high risk of developing colon cancer will allow more intensive diagnostic efforts directed toward them.

Modifications of environmental factors that are strongly implicated in the development of colon cancer represent another promising approach. It is clear that changes in dietary habits promise to go a long way toward the primary prevention of cancer of the colon.

The signs and symptoms associated with cancer of the large bowel

TABLE 7-1. SYMPTOMS ASSOCIATED WITH COLON CANCER

Abdominal pain (vague and dull)

Bleeding

Weight loss

Anemia

Change in bowel habits

Gas pains

Decrease in stool caliber

Increased use of laxatives

are variable. They will depend, to a large extent, on the size and location of the tumor within the colon. Tumors that occur on the right side of the large bowel may give rise to vague or dull abdominal pain, weight loss, or hidden bleeding. By contrast, tumors on the left side of the colon may cause gas pains, bleeding, and a decrease in stool width or caliber. Thus, there are a whole constellation of signs and symptoms associated with colon cancer (Table 7-1). If you have any of them, see your family doctor. Many patients with colon cancer delay medical care thinking these symptoms are unimportant or the result of hemorrhoids.[4,5]

RISK FACTORS IN THE DEVELOPMENT OF COLON CANCER

The relationship of nutrition to the development of colon cancer seems to be a particularly important one. Observations on the international variations in colon cancer and the striking differences in dietary patterns throughout the world raise important questions about the overall impact of nutrition in the development of cancer.

There are three postulated mechanisms by which nutritional factors are thought to play a role in the development of cancer.[6]

1. Dietary intake, including food, food additives, and possible contaminants, act as either cancer-inducing agents (carcinogens) or help to promote the development of cancer (cocarcinogens) or both.
2. Nutritional deficiencies lead to biochemical abnormalities that in some way induce cancer.
3. Excessive intake of a particular food substance produces abnormalities that lead to the development of cancer. In the particular case of colon cancer, it seems that this last mechanism is involved. Specifically, as we will discuss, dietary fat and meat consumption seem to be implicated.

In a review of the epidemiologic evidence, Wynder et al outlined the available "clues" from the world's literature that implicated nutritional influences in the development of colon cancer.[7] These findings are interesting in that they reveal the origins of the suspected association and give us some perspective on the whole issue of colon cancer. Some highlights of the review include:

1. The greatest occurrence of colon cancer is in the Western world, while the lowest rates are seen in Africa, Asia, and South America (with the exception of Argentina and Uruguay). The more developed and affluent a nation is, the greater the risk of colon cancer with the exception of Japan.

2. American blacks living in industrialized northern cities were reported to have higher colon cancer rates than blacks living in the rural South.

3. There is a higher incidence of colon cancer in American blacks compared to African blacks. Japanese immigrants to Hawaii and California have higher rates of the tumor than native Japanese. The Seventh-Day Adventists, who eat little or no meat, have a lower incidence of colon cancer than other Americans. These findings all seem to implicate environmental factors in general and diet in particular.

4. There are major differences in the rates of colon cancer between the United State and Japan and the United States and Puerto Rico. These differences correlate well with the established lower fat intake in both Japan and Puerto Rico as compared to the United States.

As a result of these and other observations, dietary factors and additional variables have been studied intensively. Factors such as constipation, weight, tobacco, and alcohol usage have shown no relationship to large bowel cancer.[8] A review of the known and suspected risk factors follows:

Dietary Fiber

The possible importance of dietary fiber on the development of colon cancer was first reported by Burkitt.[9] He noted the low colon cancer incidence and high dietary fiber intake of the South African Bantu. Higher-fiber diets result in a large stool bulk and a so-called rapid transit time. The theory is that because of the rapid transit through the colon, a cancer-inducing agent in the stool will have little time in contact with the lining of the colon; therefore, presumably, there will be little chance for the induction of tumor.

There is no general agreement on the role of dietary fiber in preventing colon cancer or, conversely, the role of a low fiber diet in promoting the disease. Dietary fiber may play a protective role in the development of colon cancer. The question remains unanswered.

Dietary Sugar

A correlation between the consumption of refined sugar and the incidence of colon cancer has been reported.[10] The author suggests that the dietary intake of refined sugar may play a causative role in the incidence of colon cancer in high-risk populations. There is evidence to dispute this association. For example, Argentina, which has a relatively high incidence of colon cancer, has a low consumption of refined sugar. Additionally, worldwide comparisons of the intake of sugar and colon cancer rates do not consistently support this relationship. At the current time, it seems doubtful that refined sugar is a risk factor in the development of colon cancer.

Dietary Fat

Many studies have demonstrated a consistent relationship between the intake of dietary animal fat and large bowel cancer.[11] There is also a similar relationship between colon cancer and meat. American diets obtain 35 to 40 percent of their fat content from beef. Therefore, the independent role of beef in the causation of colon cancer is unclear. Specific colon-cancer-inducing components of beef have not been conclusively demonstrated.

There are three current theories concerning the way in which dietary fat contributes to the development of colon cancer.[12] These include:

1. The conversion of cholesterol in the large intestines into a chemical form that is capable of inducing cancer
2. Changes in the concentrations of bile acids and activity of bacteria inside the large bowel so that cancer-producing substances are formed (Bacteria are normally found in the large bowel.)
3. Changes in the enzyme systems in the lining of the large intestines that may induce cancer

An interesting study compared samples of stool specimens from

Kuopio, Finland, and New York City.[13] Kuopio had a very low incidence of colon cancer as compared to New York, which has a high rate of colon cancer. Residents of both cities consume similar amounts of dietary fats and proteins, although the sources of fat are different. In New York, most of the fat consumption is from meat, whereas in Kuopio it is from dairy products. An analysis of the stool revealed that the fat contents were similar. However, residents of Kuopio had much bulkier quantities of stool as a result of their high intake of cereal products rich in fiber. The authors interpreted these findings to mean that the greater stool bulk diluted any cancer-causing component in the stool and prevented extensive contact of these substances with the lining of the colon. This finding would seem to add support to the role of dietary fiber in the prevention or protection against colon cancer.

There is substantial evidence that dietary fat is a risk factor in the causation of colon cancer. Precise mechanisms of action have not been delineated.

Bacterial Contents of the Bowel

No discussion of dietary influences on colon cancer development is complete without mention of the presumed role of bacteria. Bacteria are normally present in the large intestines. Most theories of the dietary etiology of colon cancer invoke these microorganisms in their rationale. They are thought to interact with the contents of the large bowel to produce cancer-inducing substances. The precise mechanism of action has not been delineated.

As one author points out, if a direct bacterial role in the etiology of the tumor is indeed proved, it could be blocked by the use of antibiotics.[14]

There are several other factors, including associated diseases, family history, and personal medical history, that are known risk factors in the development of colon cancer.[15,16]

Age

The incidence of colon cancer begins to rise slowly after the age of 40 and then takes a sharp rise at age 50. Thereafter, the risk increases with each decade of life. Men and women are at equal risk. Colon cancer can appear in young age groups, but it is usually in association with some other risk factor.

Polyps

Polyps are "cherry-like" outpouchings protruding from the lining of the large intestines. It is apparent that these can and do undergo malignant change to colon cancer. The incidence of colon cancer is higher in people with polyps or in people who have had polyps. Polyps are also known as adenomas. As an adenoma increases in size, the chance of its containing cancer increases. Thus, a 1-cm polyp has a 1 percent chance of containing cancer, a 1 to 2 cm polyp has a 10 percent chance of containing cancer, and polyps greater than 2 cm have a 30 to 50 percent rate of cancer associated with them.

The removal of these adenomas is an important part of the early detection and prevention program being advocated by many.[18,19] Removal of these growths would interrupt the chain of events whereby adenomas undergo cellular changes and become cancer.

High-Risk Groups

There are various groups of individuals who have a genetic predisposition to the development of colon cancer. Individuals with families that have a high incidence of cancer in other sites such as breast and female genital organs are at higher risk. In addition, the relatives of colon cancer patients are at three times the risk of the general population. Individuals who have had a previously cured cancer of the colon or who had polyps are at higher risk.

DISEASES ASSOCIATED WITH COLON CANCER

There are several diseases associated with the development of colon cancer.

Familial polyposis is an inherited disorder in which there are hundreds to thousands of polyps in the large bowel. These can undergo change to cancer just as any other adenoma can. The rate of development of colon cancer in these individuals is 100 percent. Surgical removal of the colon (colectomy) can prevent this.

Ulcerative colitis is a disease that involves chronic inflammation of the lining of the large bowel. Patients with long-standing ulcerative colitis are at increased risk for the development of colon cancer. The risk begins to rise after the disease is present for 7 to 10 years. After 20 years, the risk of colon cancer is 20 to 30 percent. The risk is reported to be especially high if the ulcerative colitis first appeared in an individual less than 25 years of age.

Granulomatous colitis, or so-called Crohn's disease, is also thought to place the individual at increased risk of developing colon cancer. The increased risk here is considered to be much less than that seen with ulcerative colitis.

We have noted a wide range of risk factors associated with the development of colon cancer (Tables 7-2 and 7-3). It is worthwhile to see how we can turn this information into some useful steps to decrease the death rate and disability associated with this disease.

WHAT YOU CAN DO ABOUT COLON CANCER

We mentioned in the introduction that a two-pronged approach to the prevention and successful treatment of colon cancer now seems feasible.

In the first instance, changing dietary habits seems like a very promising step in the prevention of this cancer. Available evidence indicates that you can reduce your risk, perhaps significantly, by consuming a smaller amount of dietary animal fat and adding fiber to your diet. This low-animal-fat, high-fiber diet would also be beneficial

TABLE 7-2. RISK FACTORS THAT ARE ASSOCIATED WITH THE DEVELOPMENT OF CANCER OF THE COLON

High meat intake	
High animal fat intake	
Age (more than 40 years of age)	
Associated diseases	ulcerative colitis
	granulomatous colitis
	familial polyposis syndrome
Past history	colon cancer
	polyps
	female genital or breast cancer
Family history	juvenile polyps
	colon cancer or polyps
	familial polyposis syndrome

TABLE 7-3. POSSIBLE RISK FACTORS IN THE DEVELOPMENT OF CANCER OF THE COLON

Low dietary fiber diet

High dietary intake of refined sugar

in lessening your risk of heart disease, obesity, breast cancer, and endometrial cancer. A basic dietary change is long overdue in the United States and Western countries in general. The potential benefits in health, at virtually no cost, are striking.

The second promising approach involves the early detection and treatment of colon cancer. We have noted that the poor 5-year survival is ascribed to the late stage of the disease at the time of presentation to a physician. Very often by the time symptoms have appeared, the disease is already progressed to the point where curative surgery is unlikely.

In view of the increasing occurrence of colon cancer with age, it has been advised that individuals over 40 have annual checks of their stool for blood. This is actually relatively easy to accomplish. There is available a cardboard slide with impregnated chemicals known as a "hemoccult." You simply smear a small amount of stool after each bowel movement to two slides every day for 3 days. These six slides are sent to a laboratory to test for the presence of blood. This is a very good and simple screening test that is apparently very effective in the detection of colon cancer or polyps.

In addition, it is recommended that patients over 40 have so-called sigmoidoscopy performed every 3 years. It involves the passage of a tube by a physician through the anus into the lower portion of the bowel. Some 50 percent of colon and rectal cancer can be visualized by this procedure. This technique also allows for the removal of polyps or adenomas, an important preventive measure since these growths can lead to cancer and their removal stops the process.

Individuals at high risk or individuals who have symptoms need more extensive evaluations. Procedures usually obtained at this point are the air contrast barium enema and colonoscopy. An air contrast barium enema is a radiologic procedure in which radioopaque material is introduced into the colon to obtain visualization of the lumen of the large bowel. Polyps and colon cancer as well as other pathologic conditions can be readily demonstrated. Colonoscopy is the passage of a long flexible tube known as a colonoscope into the large bowel. In the hands of a trained gastroenterologist, the entire colon and cecum (the area of the colon adjacent to the appendix) can be visualized. This is the definitive diagnosis procedure in diseases of the large bowel. Biopsies can be taken to examine tissue under a microscope, and polyps can be removed.

Colon cancer is an important example of the interaction of environment and genetics in the causation of disease. It is also an example of a disease you can do something about (Table 7-4). Change your dietary habits and get regular evaluations by your physician.

TABLE 7-4. WHAT YOU CAN DO TO LESSEN YOUR RISK OF COLON CANCER

Consume less dietary animal fat.

Eat more high fiber food.

At age 40 and older, have annual checks for blood in your stool.

At age 40 and older, have sigmoidoscopy every 3 years.

If you are in a high-risk category, have more intensive evaluations, as needed.

If you have any symptoms (Table 7-1), consult your physician immediately.

REFERENCES

1. Leffall L: Colorectal cancer — prevention and detection. *Journal of the America Cancer Society* 47:1170–1172, 1981.
2. Winawer S: Early diagnosis of colorectal cancer. *Current Concepts in Oncology*, March/April 1981, 8–6.
3. Leffall L: Colorectal cancer — prevention and detection. *Journal of the American Cancer Society* 47:1170–72, 1981.
4. Holliday H, et al: Delay in diagnosis and treatment of symptomatic colorectal cancer. *Lancet*, February 10, 1979; 309–311.
5. Pescatori M, et al: Delay in diagnosis of colorectal cancer. *Lancet*, May 26, 1979; 1137–1138.

6. Wynder E, et al: Diet and cancer of the colon. *Current Concepts in Nutrition* 6:55–71, 1977.
7. Wynder E, et al: Diet and cancer of the colon. *Current Concepts in Nutrition* 6:55–71, 1977.
8. Haskell C (ed): Cancer treatment. Philadelphia, Saunders, 1980, pp. 265–303.
9. Burkitt DP: *Cancer* 28:3, 1971.
10. Haenszel W, et al: *Journal of the National Cancer Institute* 51:1965, 1973.
11. Haskell C (ed): *Cancer Treatment.* Philadelphia, Saunders, 1980, pp 265–303.
12. Haskell C (ed): *Cancer Treatment.* Philadelphia, Saunders, 1980, pp 265–303.
13. Reddy B, et al: Fecal constituents of a high-risk North American and a low-risk Finnish population for the development of large bowel cancer. *Cancer Letters* 4:217–222, 1978.
14. Haskell C (ed): *Cancer Treatment.* Philadelphia, Saunders, 1980, pp. 265–303.
15. Winawer S: Early diagnosis of colorectal cancer. *Current Concepts in Oncology,* March/April 1981, 8–16.
16. Haskell C (ed): *Cancer Treatment,* Philadelphia, Saunders, 1980, pp 265–303.
17. Winawer S: *Early diagnosis of colorectal cancer. Current Concepts in Oncology,* March/April 1981, 8–16.
18. Leffall L: Colorectal cancer — prevention and detection. *Journal of the American Cancer Society* 47:1170–72, 1981.
19. Winawer S: Early diagnosis of colorectal cancer. *Current Concepts in Oncology,* March/April 1981, 8–16.

PART TWO

EIGHT

Smoking

Today, there can be no doubt that smoking is truly slow-motion suicide. . . .
It is nothing short of a national tragedy that so much death and disease
are wrought by a powerful habit often taken up by unsuspecting
children. . . .[1]

Joseph A. Califano, Secretary
U.S. Department of Health,
Education and Welfare

Unfortunately, there is no exaggeration in this statement. The list of
diseases causing widespread death and disability that are definitely
linked to cigarette smoking is staggering. Cigar and/or pipe smokers
face many of the same risks as cigarette smokers, although to a
somewhat lesser extent. Their risk varies, as does cigarette smokers',
with the amount of smoke that is inhaled.

It is estimated that 350,000 people will needlessly die next year
from disorders attributable to smoking.[2] From a different perspective,

139

between one-half and one-third of all cigarette smokers will die because of their smoking.[3] In 1973, the Surgeon General estimated that 4600 stillborn infants and babies who die soon after birth will be lost because of maternal smoking every year.[4] (The group of women smokers 18 to 25 is the only segment of the adult population that is increasing its smoking habit.[5])

Let's take a quick look at the consequences of this "national tragedy."

Deaths. One-quarter of U.S. deaths annually may be attributed to tobacco use.[1] The total number of deaths due to tobacco equals all the deaths from all infections (including pneumonia, influenza, and tuberculosis) plus diabetes mellitus plus all accidents (including motor vehicle) plus suicide and homicide in the United States every year.[1,6]

In other words, every year:

$$\text{Tobacco deaths} = \text{deaths from infection} + \text{diabetes} + \text{all accidents} + \text{suicide} + \text{homicide}$$

Life expectancy. It's estimated, and confirmed in many studies, that a 25-year-old man who smokes two packs a day can expect to live (on the average) 40.3 years, or until age 65, but a nonsmoker of 25 can expect to live 48.6 years, or until age 73. In other words, smoking will cost this man 8.3 years of his life.[1, 6]

Disability. The U.S. Public Health Service has calculated that every year:

- 77 million person-days are lost from work
- 88 million person-days are spent ill in bed
- There are 306 million person-days of restricted activity

These are days in excess of what would be expected if no one smoked. They are attributed directly to smoking.[1,6]

Chronic Illness. The National Clearing House for Smoking and Health estimated in 1967 that

> *... every year in the U.S. there are 11 million more chronic cases of illness. There are 280,000 more people who report a heart condition, one million more cases of chronic bronchitis and/or emphysema, 1.8 million more cases of sinusitis and one million more cases of peptic ulcer disease than there would be if no one ever smoked cigarettes.*[7]

Even if you don't succumb to the diseases known to be associated with smoking, there are still medical problems you can expect (Table 8-1).

TABLE 8-1. MORBIDITY ASSOCIATED WITH SMOKING

Smokers have:

    More coughs

    More colds

    More respiratory infections

    More shortness of breath

    More allergy problems

    Smokers take longer to recover from respiratory conditions and surgery

    Smokers lose 81 million work days more per year in the United States.

Adapted from Tobacco—Hazards to Health and Human Reproduction, Population Reports, Series L, #1, 3/79.

No matter how secure you feel, there is no doubt, if you smoke, you're at higher risk for many diseases (Table 8-2). Keep in mind that all this death and disability are completely preventable. You hold the key.

Tobacco and smoking occupy a relatively unique position in society. They are clearly as disastrous as any known epidemic, yet millions of people will quite literally "walk a mile for a Camel." Perhaps the best way to approach this paradox is from a historical perspective.[1,6,7] (Much of the information that follows was obtained from the American Cancer Society.)

Tobacco smoking was brought back to Europe by sixteenth-century Spanish explorers. Some, like Jean Nicot, French ambassador to Lisbon, thought that the tobacco leaf had beneficial medicinal effects. The tobacco plant *nicotinum tabaccum* bears his name today. There were those who as early as the 1600s saw a danger in tobacco. King James I of England in 1604 commissioned a pamphlet entitled "*A Counter Blast to Tobacco: Tobaccogenic Cancer.*" Dr. Evard, practicing

TABLE 8-2. DISEASES LINKED TO SMOKING
TOBACCO

Lung cancer

Oral cancer (Especially at risk are smokers who
drink alcohol.)

Cancer of the esophagus (Especially at risk are
smokers who drink alcohol.)

Multiple primary cancers

Laryngeal cancer (vocal cords, voice box) (Especially
at risk are smokers who drink alcohol.)

Bladder cancer (in cigarette smokers)

Kidney cancer (in cigarette smokers)

Cancer of the pancreas (in cigarette smokers)

Heart disease

Peripheral vascular disease

Bronchitis

Emphysema

Peptic ulcer disease

Cerebrovascular disease

Adverse effects during pregnancy

*Adapted from Tobacco—Hazards to Health and Human
Reproduction, Population Reports, Series L, # 1. 3/79.*

in London more than 300 years ago, said, "Tobacco causes vomit and is
an enemy of the stomach" (an apt description of nicotine toxicity even
today).

Cigarettes (paper-wrapped tobacco) were invented in Brazil in
the eighteenth century and were shipped to Spain. English troops
returning from the Crimean campaign apparently brought cigarettes
back to Britain in 1856. By 1870, the Industrial Revolution realized its
potential, and machines to make cigarettes were unfortunately invented. U.S. statistics on production first appeared in 1880. In that first
year, some 1.3 billion cigarettes were purchased (in a U.S. population of

50 million). In 1970, some 536.4 billion cigarettes were used (in a U.S. population of 204 million). By comparison, then, cigarette usage climbed 40,000 percent in the United States, while the population rose only 300 percent. In 1761, John Hill in England described cancer of the nose in snuff users. By 1795, many physicians accepted a cause and effect relationship between tobacco pipe smoking and cancer of the lower lip. The French physician Bouisson reported on a study of 68 patients with cancer of the oral cavity in 1859. He found that among 69 people with cancer of the mouth, 66 smoked tobacco, one chewed tobacco, and the others' tobacco usage was not obtainable. He also wrote that lip cancer was usually seen at the same place that the pipe or cigar was held in the mouth.

In 1927, F. R. Tylecote, a British physician, wrote that in almost every case of lung cancer he had seen or knew about, the patient was a regular smoker, most often of cigarettes. Dr. Alton Ochsner, surgeon and past president of the American Cancer Society, stated at an International Cancer Congress in 1939 that "it's our conviction that the increase in the incidence of pulmonary carcinoma (lung cancer) is due largely to the increase in smoking, particularly cigarette smoking, which is universally associated with inhalation." This link was demonstrated statistically in 1939 by Muller, who showed a strong association between cigarette smoking and lung cancer. By 1940, this relationship was widely suspected by practicing physicians.

In the 1950s, the first large-scale case-control prospective studies were carried out in England and the United States. These studies consistently showed the relationship of smoking to lung cancer and to a number of other diseases.[3,6,7] These and subsequent studies showed that the death rate among smokers from all causes was much higher than among nonsmokers. They also demonstrated relationships of smoking to heart disease, many other types of cancer, and respiratory diseases (Table 8-2).

The evidence continued to mount despite fierce opposition by the tobacco industry. On January 11, 1964, the surgeon general issued the report titled "Smoking and Health." This report took its place alongside those of Great Britain and some Scandinavian countries in their condemnation of cigarettes. Michael B. Shimuin writes in his

brilliant review of this subject: "The identification of tobacco smoking
... as a serious public health problem, ranks in importance with the
nineteenth century discoveries that polluted ground water caused
cholera and typhoid epidemics."[7]

In response to this newly defined public health danger, theCongress in 1965 passed the first national law requiring that all cigarette
packages sold within the United States bear the warning "Caution:
Cigarette smoking may be hazardous to your health." This law mandated the Federal Trade Commission (FTC) to issue annual reports on
the manufacture, promotion, and sale of cigarettes and the Department
of Health, Education and Welfare to issue reports on the relationship
between smoking and health. President Richard Nixon signed the
Public Health Smoking Act in April 1970, which made it illegal after
January 1, 1971, for cigarettes to be advertised on U.S. radio and
television.

In order to understand better how cigarette smoking can be
causally related to so many diverse pathologies, ranging from heart
disease and cancer to spontaneous abortions (miscarriages) and stillbirths, we need to take a brief look at the constituents of tobacco
smoke. An excellent recent review of tobacco and health that includes
this information is also available to health professionals.[1]

CONSTITUENTS OF TOBACCO SMOKE

There has been a great deal of research in this area. Besides the
obvious importance to medicine and interest to scientists in general,
there is a very pragmatic reason for determining the harmful components of cigarette smoke. It is one reasonable first step in the
development of a "safe" cigarette (if there is such a thing). Some
authorities feel that if we know which specific components of tobacco
smoke are harmful, we can, through various means, selectively decrease
the delivery of these substances to the smoker.

More than 4000 compounds have been isolated and identified in
tobacco smoke.[1] Tobacco smoke itself is actually a mixture of gasses
and particulate matter. Over 30 of these 4000 compounds are either
known or thought to be dangerous to your health. However, three in
particular are widely felt to be the most active agents in causing or

promoting disease: carbon monoxide, nicotine, and tar. All three are known to be toxic to humans, are found in amounts large enough to have a deleterious effect, and can readily be absorbed through the mucous membranes that they come in contact with during smoking and inhalation.

Carbon Monoxide

This colorless, odorless gas is a product of the incomplete burning of the tobacco and paper. Approximately 3 to 5 percent of cigarette smoke is carbon monoxide. A smoker who inhales receives a concentration of about 400 parts per million as compared to a nonsmoker in a smoke-filled room, who inhales concentrations of 25 to 100 parts per million. In the latter circumstance, the nonsmoker (passive smoker) is in fact being forced to inhale carbon monoxide by the smoker.

Carbon monoxide has some very interesting biochemical and physiologic features that contribute to its causative role in human illness:

1. The hemoglobin in human blood (the chemical in the body that binds oxygen so that the body can transport it to various tissues) has an attraction for the gas carbon monoxide that is 200 times stronger than its attraction for the gas oxygen.
2. The combination of hemoglobin and carbon monoxide forms a compound known as carboxyhemoglobin. This compound is unable to transport oxygen.
3. Carbon monoxide also increases the attraction of hemoglobin to oxygen that is bound to it. This results in a situation in which the hemoglobin is unable to release oxygen to the tissues it supplies.

   In other words, not only can less oxygen be taken up by the blood in the presence of carbon monoxide, but once it is taken up, it cannot as readily be released to the tissues that need it. This is thought to be the explanation of why concentrations of carboxyhemoglobin in the blood as low as 4 to 5 percent can impair the mental ability and performance of normal adults.
4. Carbon monoxide is thought to increase the formation of deposits of fatty material on the blood vessel wall, which may be a first step in "hardening of the arteries."

Nicotine

This substance is the most potent pharmacologic agent, in the concentrations present, that is found in tobacco. (In other words, nicotine elicits the greatest physiologic response or is the most powerful "drug" in tobacco smoke.) It is a thick, oily alkaloid that has no therapeutic uses. The nicotine content of tobacco varies with the type of tobacco and the form in which it is used (ie, pipe, cigar, or cigarettes and many other variables; Table 8-3). Smokers who inhale are known to retain as much as 90 percent of the nicotine content in the tobacco smoke. In the case of cigarettes, this amount will range from 0.04 mg to 3.5 mg of nicotine for each cigarette smoked.

TABLE 8-3. NICOTINE CONTENT OF TOBACCO

	Dose	Percentage by weight concentration range	
		low	*high*
Minimum dose to produce toxic symptoms	4 mg		
Fatal dose	60 mg		
Cigarettes	.04–3.5 mg per cigarette	0.9	1.96
Pipe		0.6	1.43
Cigar		0.75	3.0

Adapted from Tobacco—Hazards to Health and Human Reproduction, Population Reports, *Series L, #1. 3/79.*

It is also known that given to an individual who has not previously been receiving it, nicotine can produce toxic symptoms at a dose of only 4 mg, whereas 60 mg of nicotine given at once is a fatal dose.

Smokers of pipes and cigars who may not inhale have no reason to feel secure about the aforementioned situation. While it is true that the nicotine in cigarette smoke is absorbed mostly in the lungs, the nicotine in pipe and cigar smoke is absorbed more readily in the mouth and throat. This is true because of differences in the acid-base balance of cigarette (acidic) and pipe and cigar (alkaline) smoke.

Nicotine exerts a widespread and complex effect on many systems in the body. The drug can act as either a stimulant or relaxant on the brain. (This depends on the amount smoked and individual characteristics of the smoker.) It causes certain glands to produce stimulating hormones, adrenaline and noradrenaline (norepinephrine) and has a direct effect on the central nervous system centers that control blood pressure and heart rate.

In a normal individual, nicotine is known to have many effects:

1. It increases the heart rate, heart output, and amount of blood pumped by the heart.
2. It increases the blood pressure.
3. It increases the heart muscles need for oxygen.
4. It increases the occurrence of irregular heart rhythms (arrhythmias).
5. It increases the amount of fats in the blood (concentration of fatty acids). This may be a contributing factor in the development of arteriosclerosis (hardening of the arteries).
6. It may cause blood platelets (needed for blood clots to form) to become "stickier" and therefore clot more readily (perhaps a step in hardening of the arteries).

Carbon monoxide and nicotine acting together then team up to have a combined effect on the heart. This effect is thought to be responsible for the now firmly established link between cigarette smoking and the development of heart attacks and heart disease.[8]

On the one hand, carbon monoxide effectively reduces the amount of oxygen available to the heart at the same time as nicotine increases the heart's work and its need for oxygen. Both of these compounds are thought to play a role in arteriosclerosis, which may further narrow the blood vessels supplying the heart and therefore decrease its oxygen supply. Thus, the combination of these influences could reasonably be invoked to explain the observed causal relationship between cigarette smoking and ischemic heart disease (see Chap. 1).

Tar

Tar is the thick, dark-brown particulate material that remains after the removal of moisture and nicotine from tobacco smoke. This substance contains the compounds that are known or suspected to be cancer-causing agents (carcinogens). Agents that induce cancer are sometimes classified as "initiators" and "promoters." In this schema, it is believed that the initiators "strike first" and are "aided and abetted" by the cancer promoters. In other words, the effect of the initiator in inducing cancer is amplified and encouraged by the promoter substances. Another way of looking at this is that the initiator "prepares" the tissues for the cancer-causing effect of the promoters.

The major initiator or carcinogen found in tar is the polycyclic aromatic hydrocarbons. Stronger carcinogens such as nitrosamines and beta-naphthylamine are present in smaller amounts. Cancer promoters found in tar include the phenols and fatty acids and their esters. These substances are known to produce cancer both on direct application to the skin of test animals and when inhaled.

These three substances, tar, nicotine, and carbon monoxide, are accordingly widely believed to be responsible for the deleterious effects of cigarette smoking. Nicotine, because of its strong effect, is felt by some to be the underlying pharmacologic force behind the cigarette "habit." It has been pointed out that the rapid spread of cigarette smoking and the difficulty many people have in stopping are more characteristic of a drug dependency. The habit of smoking, however, involves many complex psychological, pharmacologic, and social factors that are intertwined.

Tobacco has now become one of the major public health hazards in the world. The 1979 U.S. Surgeon General's report on smoking and health confirms the health dangers of smoking. In that report, men who smoke cigarettes are noted to have a tenfold higher death rate for lung cancer, fivefold higher death rate for bronchitis, emphysema, and asthma and a two- to threefold greater death rate from heart disease than men who do not smoke. The risk of death increases progressively with the amount smoked.[1]

TOBACCO AND LUNG CANCER

Since the early association of smoking cigarettes with lung cancer in 1927 by Tylecote and the first studies begun in the 1950s, the evidence has been overwhelming. All studies, both prospective (a "forward looking" study in which a population is studied over a period of time) and retrospective (a review of a population and their history "backward looking") have consistently shown a strong linkage between smoking cigarettes and lung cancer. The increase in mortality from lung cancer has (as would be expected) skyrocketed along with the use of cigarettes after World War II. In the United States the lung cancer death rates increased fivefold between 1945 and 1975. This has been called an "alarming epidemic" by the U.S. Public Health Service. It is also estimated that in the next 10 years (due to the increase in women smokers) lung cancer will exceed breast cancer as the major cause of death from cancer in U.S. women.[1]

Cigarette smokers face a death rate from lung cancer that ranges from 8 to 15 times that of people who have never smoked. This link between smoking and lung cancer is especially strong for the oat cell and squamous cell types of lung tumor but holds true for all types. It is variously estimated that smoking is responsible for 80 to 90 percent of all lung tumors. Lung cancer has a uniformly poor prognosis, with a fatal outcome more than 90 percent of the time. The death rate for cigar and/or pipe smokers from lung cancer varies from two to six times that found in nonsmokers.[7] (In this situation as in the other diseases associated with smoking, we are apparently dealing with a dose-response situation. In other words, the larger the dose, that is, the more inhaled quantity smoked, etc, the more likely the development of disease.)

There is a great deal of evidence that suggests that there are progressive cellular changes that occur before the development of cancer. In other words, before the onset of malignant change to cancer (and its presumed irreversible nature), there are many smaller changes (and therefore potentially reversible ones) that occur. In fact, this seems to be borne out. A prospective British trial conducted by the Royal College of Physicians on 34,490 doctors yielded some interesting data.[7] This study followed a large group who markedly decreased their cigarette smoking in the period 1954–1965. The lung cancer mortality rate among British doctors declined by 38 percent in this period at the same time as the rate for all men in England and Wales (who did not change their smoking habits) increased by 7 percent.

The beneficial effects of the cessation of smoking have been borne out in other studies.[7] The lessening of risk increases with the amount of time the smoker has stopped. Even if you have smoked heavily for many years, you can anticipate a marked reduction in risk of lung cancer after 10 years. Ex-smokers of less than one pack per day

show a reduced mortality rate as early as 1 to 4 years after stopping.
There are other known carcinogens in the environment that can cause lung cancer. However, the risk to the smoker who is also exposed to these carcinogens is greatly multiplied. If you smoke and your job brings you into contact with these agents, you are at high risk of developing lung cancer (Table 8-4).

TABLE 8-4. SMOKING TOBACCO AND OCCUPATIONAL EXPOSURES AT HIGH RISK FOR LUNG CANCER

Cigarette smoking

   +

Uranium miners

Asbestos workers

People who work with:
   arsenic
   chromium
   nickel
   coal
   natural gas
   graphite

   =

Greatly increased risk for the development of lung cancer

Adapted from Tobacco—Hazards to Health and Human Reproduction, Population Reports, Series L, #1. 3/79.

TOBACCO AND ORAL CANCER

Smoking tobacco plays a causative role in the development of cancers of the oral cavity. Most cancers of the mouth are rare in nonsmokers. The cancer-causing effect of tobacco smoke in this disease is exacerbated, as in cancer of the larynx (voice box) and esophagus by alcohol intake. One explanation for the apparent potentiation of the effect of tobacco smoke by alcohol is that the alcohol carries the tar (where it is believed the carcinogenic activity resides) into contact with the membranes lining the mouth and throat. The association of alcohol and tobacco in producing oral cancer has recently been demonstrated in women.[9]

Cigar and pipe smoking has been reported to be as dangerous as cigarette smoking in oral cancer. The risk of death from oral cancer is three- to tenfold greater among cigarette smokers and three- to fivefold greater among pipe and cigar smokers.

TOBACCO AND CANCER OF THE ESOPHAGUS

Cigarette, cigar, and/or pipe smokers have a two- to sixfold greater death rate from cancer of the esophagus than nonsmokers. The likelihood of developing cancer increases both with the amount of tobacco smoked and the amount of alcohol consumed.

This tumorlike cancer of the oral cavity and larynx (voice box) expresses itself more readily when tobacco smoke and alcohol act in combination.

TOBACCO AND CANCER OF THE LARYNX

Cancer of the larynx (voice box, or vocal cords) is rare among non-smokers. This tumor can be divided into intrinsic and extrinsic cancer of the larynx. The intrinsic tumor or cancer of the "true" vocal cords is associated with smoking and has no relationship to alcohol intake. The extrinsic tumor acts in a manner similar to oral and esophageal cancer, that is, it expresses itself more frequently in the presence of alcohol. Statistics for the two different lesions are not kept separately. Laryngeal cancer, both intrinsic and extrinsic, is considered statistically as one entity. Therefore, this lesion does show a relationship to smoking and alcohol acting together. The mortality rate from laryngeal cancer increased six- to tenfold among cigarette smokers and three- to tenfold among cigar and/or pipe smokers compared to nonsmokers.

TOBACCO AND BLADDER CANCER

There is an apparent association between bladder cancer and cigarette smoking. This link is not as strong as that seen in the previously discussed tumors. Cigarette smokers face a death rate from bladder cancer, which is two- to threefold greater than that seen in nonsmokers. One investigator estimated that 39 percent of the male bladder cancer cases and 29 percent of the female cases are related to cigarette smoking.[7]

There is no proven relationship between cigar and/or pipe smoking and bladder cancer at present.

TOBACCO AND CANCER OF THE KIDNEY

Cancer of the kidney has also been linked to cigarette smoking. Cigarette smokers have a twofold greater risk of death from the tumor than nonsmokers.

One possible explanation for cancer of the pelvis and of the kidney and bladder is the hypothesized presence of carcinogens from tobacco smoke in the urine of smokers. Others have reported an aberration of tryptophan (an amino acid) metabolism in cigarette smokers. In this view, the tryptophan metabolites such as hydroxyanthranilic acid and hydroxykynurenine are carcinogenic.

TOBACCO AND CANCER OF THE PANCREAS

Cancer of the pancreas has an established relationship to cigarette smoking. There may be an association between cigar smoking and this devastating cancer as well. Cigarette smokers have a twofold increased death rate from cancer of the pancreas compared to nonsmokers.

Wynder et al have offered a very interesting hypothesis for the mechanism of carcinogensis in this tumor.[7] In their view, carcinogens from tobacco smoke and occupational exposures are excreted into the bile. Through the mechanism of reflux or (backflow) into the pancreatic duct and with possible interaction of bile acids and the metabolites of cholesterol, there begins the process of malignant change.

TOBACCO AND HEART DISEASE

There is a very well established relationship between smoking tobacco and ischemic heart disease and heart attacks. A recently published 11-year study of 4004 men and women, which adjusted for 48 possible interactions, demonstrated this powerful link.[10] In that study, the mortality rate from heart disease was 3.6 to 4.7 times greater for cigarette smokers than nonsmokers. There is a definite, but smaller, increased risk for cigar and/or pipe smokers as well.

More Americans die from heart disease than any other health

problem in the United States. The possible explanations for the increased risk faced by smokers have been discussed in the section on tobacco smoke constituents.

The risk of heart disease is directly related to the number of cigarettes smoked and the duration of smoking. It is estimated that 37 percent of the "excess" deaths caused by cigarette smoking are due to heart disease.[8] This risk is reportedly substantially reduced when cigarette smoking is stopped.[8] Many studies confirm the important role cigarette smoking plays in the occurrence of heart attacks and heart disease.[11,12] In the previously discussed prospective study of British doctors who stopped smoking, it was found that the mortality rate from heart disease in this group fell 6 percent, while the rate for the male population as a whole rose 9 percent.[3]

It should be noted that women who smoke and take birth control pills are at a particularly increased risk for both heart attacks and strokes[13,14] (Table 8-5). It has even been proposed that smoking be a contraindication to the use of birth control pills.

TABLE 8-5. SMOKING TOBACCO AND ENVIRONMENTAL EXPOSURES PRODUCING HIGH RISK

Alcohol consumption (increased cancer risk)
Women using birth control pills (increased stroke risk and heart attack risk)
Occupational exposures (Table 8-4)
Presence of known risk factors for heart attacks (eg, high blood pressure, high cholesterol, obesity, inactivity)

Adapted from Tobacco—Hazards to Health and Human Reproduction, Population Reports, Series L, #1. 3/79.

TOBACCO AND STROKES

There is reportedly an association between cigarette smoking and stroke. In the age range 45 to 54, male smokers had a death rate 50 to 100 percent higher than that of nonsmokers.[6] A California study of 17,939 women showed that women smokers had a risk 5.7 times that of nonsmokers.[14] In women who smoked and used birth control pills, the risk leaped to 22 times that of nonsmokers.

TOBACCO AND RESPIRATORY DISEASES

Deaths from pulmonary emphysema and chronic bronchitis in the United States have risen (similar to the lung cancer situation) since 1945. In that year, 2666 deaths were reported from chronic bronchitis and emphysema whereas in 1968 the number was 30,390, 11 times as great.[6]

A prospective study of British physicians found that deaths from chronic bronchitis and emphysema were directly related to the amount of cigarettes smoked.[3] In that study, mortality from bronchitis was seen 20 times more often among those smoking 25 or more cigarettes a day as compared to nonsmokers. Among these physicians as a group, many of whom stopped smoking, the death rate from bronchitis fell 22 percent between the 1950s and 1960s compared to a drop of 4 percent for the male population as a whole. The surgeon general reported that in seven large prospective studies involving almost 2 million people in several countries, the mortality rate for chronic bronchitis and emphysema was more than six times as great as that observed in nonsmokers.[6]

Some apt descriptions help demonstrate the horrors of chronic lung disease:[6] "The person who gets lung cancer from smoking is lucky in comparison to the person who gets emphysema, because lung cancer is usually of short duration, while patients with emphysema spend years of their lives gasping and struggling for breath."

The American Cancer Society booklet describes a person with emphysema: "He is exhausted all the time; gasping like a fish out of water."

An interesting study of the interrelationship of symptoms of lung disease and smoking habits was recently done.[15] In that study, most male smokers who developed lung disease quit because of symptoms of the disease, whereas it is noted that ex-smokers with diagnosed disease had fewer symptoms.

TOBACCO AND PREGNANCY

Smoking cigarettes by pregnant women has now been shown to be hazardous to the unborn child and contributes to complications of pregnancy and labor (Table 8-6). Early research on tobacco smoking

TABLE 8-6. SMOKING DURING PREGNANCY; ADVERSE EFFECTS OF TOBACCO

Lower birth weights (Lower than normal birth weight is associated with a child's poor physical and emotional development.)

Shortened gestation (premature delivery)

Higher rates of spontaneous abortion (miscarriages, especially in the last months of pregnancy)

More frequent complications of pregnancy and labor

Higher rates of perinatal mortality (increased still births and increased mortality among newborns)

Adapted from Tobacco—Hazards to Health and Human Reproduction, Population Reports, *Series L, #1. 3/79.*

focused on adult males. However, with the increase in women smokers (as noted previously, the FTC reports that in 1978 young women smokers from 18 to 25 were the only segment of the adult population that increased their habit), more attention was focused on this group, and the effects of smoking during pregnancy were associated with lower birth weights, shortened length of pregnancy (gestation), higher rates of spontaneous abortions (miscarriages), more frequent complications of pregnancy and labor, and, most loathsome, higher rates of stillborns and newborn deaths.[1, 16-19] There is some suggestion of an association between smoking and congenital malformations (birth defects) as well.[20]

In a review of this problem it has been estimated that for a healthy young women who receives good prenatal care and is a moderate smoker, the risk of having a child with a birth defect is 10 to 20 percent greater than for a nonsmoker. However, in a heavy smoker who is older, poor, or anemic, the risk of a miscarriage or newborn death is 100 percent higher than in a nonsmoker. Carbon monoxide and nicotine are the agents in tobacco smoke thought to be responsible.[1]

The dangers of cigarette smoking to the infant may not stop at birth. Infants who are breastfed by mothers who smoke will consume nicotine and possibly DDT. Infants in families in which a parent smokes are thought to be more at risk of developing bronchitis or pneumonia during their first year. Finally, the notorious Sudden Infant Death Syndrome (SID) may be more prevalent in families in which the mother smokes.[1]

It is clear that smoking cigarettes is a real danger to the unborn child and possibly the mother (increased complications of pregnancy). Smoking cigarettes has been reported to be associated with an early change of life (menopause)[21] and may be linked to cancer of the cervix.[22]

THE ECONOMICS OF TOBACCO

No disccusion of tobacco is complete without a brief look at the economic "advantages" of cancer. Tobacco is an important crop in 16 states and is particularly important in the agriculture of North Carolina and Kentucky. The manufacture and distribution of tobacco are controlled by large multinational corporations. They contribute positively to the economy in two basic ways:

1. They are heavily taxed and in 1977 yielded $6.2 billion in taxation revenues to the government.
2. As an exported product, they make a sizable contribution to the balance of trade. In 1977, U.S. consumers spent $17 billion, which yielded $10.8 billion income and taxes of $6.2 billion. It is estimated that total consumer spending including exports, is about $19.6 billion, and the tobacco industry supports jobs for 1.3 million people.

These advantages must be weighed against the economic cost to society in terms of lost production from illness, cost of health care, and loss of life and property from illness and fire. One estimate of these costs is $27.5 billion. Thus, the cost to society in real economic terms is greater than the alleged economic benefit. (Nowhere in these calculations is there, or could there be, a "cost" in dollars of the human anguish and suffering that results.)

These estimates and much of the data were obtained from the information pamphlet *Tobacco-Hazards to Health and Reproduction.*[1]

PREVENTION AND YOU

Smoking tobacco is a real danger and is implicated in a broad spectrum of diseases ranging from heart disease and cancer to newborn deaths. Many agencies, both semigovernmental and voluntary, have been notable in their fight against this hazard. The American Cancer Society has led the way since the early association of lung cancer and cigarette smoking. Between 1955 and 1968, the percentage of adult men who smoke declined from 53 percent to 38 percent. Adult women who regularly smoke rose from 25 percent to 32 percent between 1955 and 1965; however, from 1965 to 1978, it fell back to 30 percent. The percentage of all adults who were regular smokers in 1978 was only 33 percent, the lowest in more than 30 years. Women aged 18 to 25 were the only segment of the adult population in whom smoking was increasing.[5]

The challenge to government, society, and you is clear. It is not easy to stop smoking, but it's estimated that more than 30 million Americans have stopped smoking. There are many programs, both commercial and voluntary, that are available to help. These programs can take many varied forms.[7]

Physical counseling

It has been estimated that a simple, firm admonition from your doctor can result in 10 percent of smokers stopping and staying off cigarettes.

Hypnosis

There are several ways in which hypnosis can be used to help smokers stop. There can be one or several sessions. Techniques differ and can utilize the posthypnotic suggestion that cigarettes taste bad or emphasize more positive aspects of the smoker's quitting. Sometimes the smoker is taught self-hypnosis as a relaxation technique and "built in" reinforcement. Initial success rates are very high, with tapering off following treatment. Long-term results have been reported to yield a success rate between 20 to 40 percent. The lower figure is probably more accurate.

Group Counseling

This is a well-accepted approach to aid smokers in quitting. In most situations, groups of 10 to 20 smokers will meet for a series of discussions on smoking. Sometimes groups are led by an ex-smoker who can offer suggestions. The American Cancer Society offers "Quit Smoking Clinics" in many areas that utilize this approach. Typical of these clinics is eight sessions over a 2-week period. This is a fairly effective method, with long-term success rates reported at 20 to 25 percent. It has been suggested that prolonged follow-up activities can improve the long-term success rate to 50 percent.[23]

Drug Treatment and Conditions

These treatments have not been very successful. They are of interest primarily because of their unique approaches. In the drug treatment approach, the habit of cigarette smoking is considered to be largely a drug dependency on nicotine. In order to help the smoker quit and to avoid "withdrawal," a drug with properties similar to nicotine is prescribed. It has been found that it offered no advantage over a placebo (sugar pill), and any effectiveness in this modality was probably the result of physician counseling that accompanied the drug.

The conditioning programs try to replace smoking cigarettes with a negative or painful feeling. Forcing smokers to face smoke-blowing machines or using electric shocks when he lights up a cigarette are techniques that have been used. These approaches have not proved very successful.

Many smokers are able to quit on their own. The American Cancer Society has available a "tip sheet" with some 40 different aids to stop smoking. Some aids that have been suggested appear promising (Table 8-7).[24,25] Among these aids, there are some very ingenious ideas. However, on the lighter side, there are also some peculiar ones.[25]

TABLE 8-7. HELPFUL HINTS TO STOP SMOKING

1. List the reasons for and against smoking.

2. Change to a low-tar, low-nicotine brand.

3. Select a day to quit.

4. Chart your smoking habits for two weeks: how many cigarettes, when, which is the most and least important?

5. Each night repeat at least ten times one of your reasons for not smoking.

6. Eliminate one cigarette from your routine: the most or least desired.

7. Quit on the day you selected. Keep busy: go to the movies, exercise, take long walks. Use substitutes: sip water, chew gum, eat raisins or carrots, chew a clove.

Adapted from Strong.[24]

#15: Put away your ashtrays or fill them with objects so they cannot be used for ashes. Plant flowers in them or fill them with walnuts. The latter will give you something to do with your hands.

#24: Take a shower. You cannot smoke in the shower.

#40: Give yourself time to think and get fit by walking one-half hour each day. If you have a dog, take him for a walk with you.

Stopping your smoking habit is a very important issue to you personally. There is evidence to suggest that if you stop smoking, your risk for a heart attack rapidly falls, perhaps immediately.[23] It's important for you, your family, and the ones you love. Do something about it now for them and for you.

> *Tobacco is a filthy weed,*
> *That from the devil does proceed*
> *It drains your purse, it burns your clothes,*
> *And makes a chimney of your nose.*
> *Oliver Wendell Holmes[1]*
> *(1809–1894)*

REFERENCES

1. *Tobacco — Hazards to Health and Human Reproduction. Population Reports* Ser L, no. 1, 1979.
2. Fishman A: How Safe Can Cigarettes Be? *New England Journal of Medicine*, 1979.
3. Doll R: Mortality in relation to smoking: 20 years of observations on male British doctors. *British Medical Journal* 1976.
4. Fielding J: Smoking and pregnancy. Massachusetts Department of Public Health, 298: 1978.
5. Ask Tax Dollars to Light An Antismoking Fire. *Daily News,* December, 1979.
6. *The Dangers of Smoking—The Benefits of Quitting.* American Cancer Society, 1977, p. 19.
7. Schottenfeld D: *Cancer Epidemiology and Prevention,* American Cancer Society.
8. Revised ad hoc Comittee Report on Cigarette Smoking and Cardiovascular Disease. American Heart Association 1977.

9. Bross I: Early onset of oral cancer among women who drink and smoke. *Oncology* 33:136–139, 1976.
10. Friedman G, et al: Mortality in middle-aged smokers and nonsmokers. *New England Journal of Medicine* 300: 1979.
11. Bergstrand R, et al: Myocardial infarction among men below age 40. *British Heart Journal* 783–788, 1978.
12. Dick TBS, et al: Prevalence of three major risk factors in random sample of men and women, and in patients with ischaemic heart disease, *British Heart Journal*, 617–626, 1978.
13. Jain A: Cigarette smoking, use of oral contraceptives, and myocardial infarction. *American Journal of Obstetrics and Gynecology* 126: 1976.
14. Petitti D, et al: Use of oral contraceptives, cigarette smoking, and risk of subarachnoid hemmorhage. *Lancet*, 1978.
15. Lebowitz M: Smoking habits and changes in smoking habits as they relate to chronic conditions and respiratory symptoms. *American Journal of Epidemiology* 105: 1977.
16. Fielding J: Smoking and Pregnancy, *Massachusetts Department of Public Health* 298: 1978.
17. Silverman D: Maternal smoking and birth weight. *American Journal of Epidemiology* 105: 1977.
18. Meyer M, et al: Perinatal events associated with maternal smoking during pregnancy. *American Journal of Epidemiology* 103: 1976.
19. Kline J, et al: Smoking: a risk factor for spontaneous abortion. *New England Journal of Medicine* 297: 1977.
20. Kelsey J, et al: Maternal smoking and congenital malformations: an epidemiological study. *Journal of Epidemiologic and Community Health* 102–07, 1978.
21. Jick H, et al: Relation between smoking and age of natural menopause. *Lancet* 1977.
22. Winkelstein W: Smoking and cancer of the uterine cervix: hypothesis *American Journal of Epidemiology* 106: 1977.
23. Wynder E, et al: Tobacco and Health. *The New England Journal of Medicine* 1979.
24. Strong J, et al: Cigarette smoking and atherosclerosis in autopsied men. *Atherosclerosis* 23:451–476, 1976.
25. American Cancer Society Tip Sheet.

NINE

Obesity

"Obesity, defined as an excessive accumulation of body fat is one of the most common and most puzzling disorders of modern times."[1]

It has been noted that the ease with which humans can store energy in the form of body fat has been a major factor in the survival of our species. In areas of the world in which the food supply is inconsistent or occasionally unreliable, these fat stores continue to be important in daily survival. However, in Western societies where both a wide variety and quantity of food is consistently available, the only constrictions on consumption are personal traits and custom. The result has been a virtual epidemic of obesity and diets rich in animal protein and cholesterol, all of which are known to be associated with a shortened life expectancy. Obesity is an increasing problem for all the countries of the Western world.[5]

A review of actuarial data summarizing the experiences of 5 million people insured by 26 life insurance companies revealed that 30 percent of men and 40 percent of women between the ages of 40 and 49 are at least 20 percent above their ideal weights as established by the Metropolitan Life Insurance Co. (Tables 9-1 and 9-2).[4] Ideal weight is defined as the weight group with the lowest mortality for a given height. The prevalence of obesity is even greater with advancing age, decreasing socioeconomic levels, and in certain ethnic groups.[5] Children are even at risk. Ten to 15 percent of young children are obese. This cannot be lightly ignored as "baby fat"; 80 percent of these children become obese adults with all the physical and emotional perils that entails.[5] It is apparent from the above that obesity is a major health problem in the United States.

An obese individual has an abnormally high accumulation of body fat. This disorder is the most common metabolic abnormality in areas of the world in which the food supply is abundant. The accumulation of fat occurs when the caloric intake in the diet supplies more energy than the body can utilize in physical activity and growth. The excess energy, in the form of fat, is stored in so-called adipose tissue.

Several procedures and standards have been developed to quantify more objectively degrees of body fatness. Simpler methods include observation, the use of height and weight tables, and measurements of skin-fold thickness. More sophisticated and theoretically more accurate measures include the use of densitometry, which consists of weighing an individual in and out of water. From the differences in weights and a knowledge of the relative density of fat and lean body mass, the fat fraction can be calculated. Other techniques utilize radioactive isotopes of potassium. From a realistic perspective, height and weight tables and measurements of skin-fold thickness are widely used and considered an accurate measure of obesity.

Obesity has been associated with a great many serious medical problems, including high blood pressure, diabetes mellitus, breast cancer, endometrial cancer, multiple complications, and many others. There is an important association between obesity and the development of heart disease. It has been estimated that if every American were at ideal weight, there would be 25 percent less heart disease and 35 percent fewer episodes of stroke and heart failure.[7]

Physical illness is not the only deleterious consequence of obesity. As one behavioral scientist notes:[8] "The psychological perils of obesity can be far-ranging, disabling and permanent." Preoccupation with

TABLE 9-1. WEIGHTS FOR MEN OF AGES 25 AND OVER

| Desirable Weight in Pounds According to Frame (in indoor clothing) | | | | | 50% Over Desirable Weight | | | | |
| Height (with shoes on) (1-in heels) | | Small Frame | Medium Frame | Large Frame | Height (with shoes on) (1-in heels) | | Small Frame | Medium Frame | Large Frame |
Feet	Inches				Feet	Inches			
5	2	112–120	118–129	126–141	5	2	180	193	211
5	3	115–123	121–133	129–144	5	3	184	199	216
5	4	118–126	124–136	132–148	5	4	189	204	222
5	5	121–129	127–139	135–152	5	5	193	208	228
5	6	124–133	130–143	138–156	5	6	199	214	234
5	7	128–137	134–147	142–161	5	7	205	220	241
5	8	132–141	138–152	147–166	5	8	211	228	249
5	9	136–145	142–156	151–170	5	9	217	234	250
5	10	140–150	146–160	155–174	5	10	225	240	261
5	11	144–154	150–165	159–179	5	11	231	244	268
6	0	148–158	154–170	164–184	6	0	237	255	276
6	1	152–162	158–175	168–189	6	1	243	262	283
6	2	156–167	162–180	173–194	6	2	250	270	291
6	3	160–171	167–185	178–199	6	3	256	277	298
6	4	164–175	172–190	182–204	6	4	262	285	306

Source: Metropolitan Life Insurance Company.

TABLE 9-2. WEIGHTS FOR WOMEN OF AGES 25 AND OVER

| Desirable Weight in Pounds According to Frame (in Indoor Clothing) | | | | | 50% Over Desirable Weight* | | | |
| Height (with shoes on) (1-in heels) | | Small Frame | Medium Frame | Large Frame | Height (with shoes on) (1-in heels) | | Small Frame | Medium Frame | Large Frame |
Feet	Inches				Feet	Inches			
4	10	92–98	96–107	104–119	4	10	147	160	178
4	11	94–101	98–110	106–122	4	11	151	165	183
5	0	96–104	101–113	109–125	5	0	156	169	187
5	1	99–107	104–116	112–128	5	1	160	174	192
5	2	102–110	107–119	115–131	5	2	165	178	196
5	3	105–113	110–122	118–134	5	3	169	183	201
5	4	108–116	113–126	121–138	5	4	174	189	207
5	5	111–119	116–130	125–142	5	5	178	195	213
5	6	114–123	120–135	129–146	5	6	184	202	219
5	7	118–127	124–139	133–150	5	7	190	208	225
5	8	122–131	128–143	137–154	5	8	196	214	231
5	9	126–135	132–147	141–158	5	9	202	220	237
5	10	130–140	136–151	145–163	5	10	210	226	244
5	11	134–144	140–155	149–168	5	11	216	232	252
6	0	138–148	144–159	153–173	6	0	222	238	259

Source: Metropolitan Life Insurance Company
*For girls between 18 and 25, subtract 1 lb. for each year under 25.

weight, psychological and sexual maladjustment, and poor body image have all been reported.

The process of dieting itself can be very stressful from a psychological perspective.[9] There is intense and unremitting social pressure from family, friends, and peers to lose weight. The obese individual thus can initiate a lifelong process of short-lived diet success followed by failure and weight gain with a resultant sense of guilt and loss of self-esteem. This cycle of failure can cause depression, anxiety, irritability, and other emotional disturbances.

"Millions are plagued by excess weight. Many attempt to reduce by methods that are largely ineffective. Confronted by failure, they move on to another approach and then another, creating a lucrative market for those who promote what cannot be delivered. The fact that so many overweight people are attracted to questionable measures is testimony to how desperately they want to lose weight and how difficult it is for them to do so. Millions more have given up even trying."[10]

OBESITY AS A RISK FACTOR

For many years, obesity and weight gain have been associated with illness and untimely death. Mortality statistics show a reduction in life expectancy with obesity even when this is of moderate degree, that is, 10 percent to 20 percent overweight.[11] Men 10 percent or more overweight had an increase in mortality of 33 percent, while those who were 20 percent or more overweight had a nearly 50 percent increase in death rate.[12]

There are a great many physical and mental disorders linked to obesity (Tables 9-3 and 9-4). A review of the evidence that associates obesity with several serious diseases will serve to place into perspective the detrimental effects of obesity in our society.

OBESITY AND HEART DISEASE

There have been consistent and reliable data showing that obesity is associated with the development of ischemic heart disease.[13-16] It appears that this effect of excess weight on heart disease is mediated through exacerbation of other known risk factors. In other words, obesity is known to elevate blood pressure, raise blood lipids (fat

TABLE 9-3. DISEASES COMMONLY ASSOCIATED WITH OBESITY

High blood pressure

Heart disease

Stroke

Gall bladder disease

Diabetes mellitus (sugar diabetes)

Cancer of the breast and endometrium

Hiatal hernia

Psychiatric conditions

Increased surgical risk

Kidney disease

Gout

TABLE 9-4. PSYCHOLOGICAL IMPAIRMENT ASSOCIATED WITH OBESITY

Impairment of self-image with feelings of inferiority

Social isolation

Subject to social, economic, and other types of discrimination

Neuroses

Loss of mobility

Increased employee absenteeism

Adapted from Van Itallie.[13]

levels), and increase the blood sugar levels (a tendency toward sugar diabetes). These are all known risk factors in heart disease.

Data from the large prospective Framingham Study clearly show that obese people are more likely to develop heart disease.[17,18] They have shown that for every 10 percent increase in weight, there is a 6.5-mm increase in systolic blood pressure, a 12-mg/dl rise in plasma cholesterol, and a 2-mg/dl rise in fasting blood sugar. The authors of this report, Gordon and Kannel, point out a potential source of optimism in these findings:[19]

> *Because it reversibly promotes atherogenic traits like hypertension, diabetes and hyperlipidemia (high blood fats), reduction of overweight is probably the most important hygienic measure (aside from avoidance of cigarettes) available for the control of cardiovascular disease. In other words, the loss of weight can reverse the elevation of risk factors associated with obesity and lessen your chances of heart disease.*

OBESITY AND DIABETES MELLITUS

There is a well-known association with excessive body weight and the development of adult onset diabetes mellitus.[20] This relationship has been shown in both cross-cultural and prospective studies. Although heart disease is responsible for the greatest increase in death rate among obese people, diabetes is responsible for the greatest relative increase in mortality in association with degrees of fatness. In a prospective study, it was shown that in moderate obesity the risk of diabetes was increased ten times, whereas in those 45 percent or more overweight, the risk of diabetes was thirty-fold.[21]

OBESITY AND HIGH BLOOD PRESSURE

Several large prospective studies have demonstrated an association between obesity and high blood pressure.[22–24] This is a real association and not, as previously thought, related to artifacts incurred in taking the blood pressure of obese patients. High blood pressure is a known risk factor in several major diseases, including heart attacks and strokes. Weight loss can be expected to reverse the component of high blood pressure associated with obesity.

OBESITY AND GALL BLADDER DISEASE

There are several sources of data that demonstrate that obesity is associated with gallstones. Evidence from prospective studies, postmortem examinations, and case-report analysis consistently support this relationship.[25,26] Within any given age group, the prevalence of gall bladder disease increases with the degree of obesity.[27]

Gallstones may require surgical removal. It has been pointed out that obesity increases the risks of surgery.[28] Thus, one risk factor, obesity, can both necessitate surgery and increase its risks.

OBESITY AND MUSCULOSKELETAL DISORDERS

There is an association between obesity and osteoarthritis. This has been seen in particular in the knees and other weight-bearing joints. It is also believed that obesity may exacerbate preexisting postural problems.

OBESITY AND THE RISKS OF SURGERY

Obese people are generally believe to face greater problems at surgery and in the postoperative period. Obesity makes surgery more difficult from a technical point of view. Overweight people are more likely to experience problems such as wound separations or infection and the development of blood clots on the lungs.[29,30]

OBESITY AND CANCER

Obesity has been linked to breast cancer, colon cancer, and cancer of the endometrium.[31, 32] Many authors have suggested weight reduction as well as diets lower in animal fat as possible steps toward the prevention of these diseases.

TABLE 9-5. FACTORS THAT MAY PREDISPOSE TO THE DEVELOPMENT OF OBESITY

Aging (with an accompanying fall in metabolic rate)

Decreased physical activity

Family and cultural eating habits

Depression or anxiety

Childhood obesity

We have noted that obesity is linked to a great many varied physical and mental disorders that affect mankind. Despite these known associations, obesity remains widespread in Western societies. An overview of some of the factors that lead to obesity may give added insight into the problem (Table 9-5).

FACTORS LINKED TO THE DEVELOPMENT OF OBESITY

Family and cultural eating patterns are considered important in the development of obesity. Cultural patterns that place emphasis on eating can imbue food with psychologic significance, making it a source of gratification that may be unrelated to hunger or nutritional needs. Certain cultures equate success with obesity.

Psychological factors are thought to be of significance in overeating. In this view, food is used as a substitute for sources of gratification that might ordinarily be derived from friends, family, or job satisfaction. Depression or anxiety can also be manifested by overeating. In this case, the resultant obesity can only serve to increase isolation and worsen the original psychological need.

It is known that a high percentage of overweight children become overweight adults.[33,34] There have been several studies designed to elucidate what the risk factors were for the development of obesity in these children. In one study of overweight children, several factors were isolated.[35] These included: obesity in a first-degree relative (mother, father, sister, or brother), an elderly mother, being an only child, and the absence of one parent. Two or more of these factors were present in sixty percent of the obese children studied. Another study found that physically inactive children, especially from low socioeconomic levels, were at particular risk.[36]

Obesity in children is a serious problem. In youth, it is a source of poor self-image and feelings of low esteem often accompanied by individual and peer rejection and isolation. As an adult, it can lead to all the physical disease and impairment already discussed. "Baby fat" is not cute, and it is the minority of children that can be expected to "grow out of it."

THE TREATMENT OF OBESITY

Protein Diet Supplements

The prolonged use of starvation or severe dietary restriction supplemented by "liquid protein" has been shown to be very dangerous and sometimes deadly. Fifty-eight deaths were reported in the late 1970s in association with individuals utilizing starvation and "predigested liquid protein" products. These products contain hydrolysates of collagen, which are of very low biologic value. The Food and Drug Administration (FDA) in conjunction with the Center on Disease Control studied these deaths. Seventeen obese but otherwise healthy women were found to have died of irregular heart rhythms.[37]

Thyroid Medication

There is no place for the use of thyroid medication in the management of obesity. Large doses of this medication may cause irregular heart rhythms and heart failure. When used in combination with amphetamines or water pills, these drugs are particularly dangerous.

Amphetamines

Amphetamines and their derivatives induce a feeling of "well-being" and through this mechanism modify patterns of overeating. There is rapid tolerance to the use of these drugs. In other words, after a period of time, it takes more medication to produce the same behavioral effect. These drugs have a high risk of habituation. In addition, any weight loss that results is almost always of a very transient nature.

Behavior Modification

Behavior therapy is a new and relatively promising approach to the problem of obesity. The major premise underlying these programs is that significant changes in both eating and exercise behavior is necessary to ensure long-term weight control. The major features of such a program have recently been outlined.[38] These include:

Self-monitoring. Patients are encouraged to keep records of food intake, calories, factors that influence eatihg, physical activity, and body weight.

Stimulus control. Obese people have been shown to be highly responsive to food "cues" such as palatibility of food, time of day, and physical location (eg, in the kitchen). Patients are taught to limit their access to food, using shopping lists, and to eliminate food displays such as candy, nut dishes, and cookie jars.

Slow eating
Slowing the process of eating will allow the absorption of nutrients to occur while the meal is still being eaten. This will help produce early feelings of satiety. Simply putting the fork down between bites is a mechanical step that can reinforce such behavior.

Nutritional Education
Nutritional counseling to help obese individuals understand their real nutritional needs is an important part of the program. The relationship between overeating, caloric intake, and obesity is discussed.

Exercise
This is an important feature in a weight-control program. There are substantial benefits to be accrued through exercise in addition to the expenditures of calories involved in the activity. Evidence indicates that physical activity may actually reduce appetite in a sedentary individual. It is also known that exercise increases the metabolic rate for long periods after the actual act of physical exertion.

Reinforcement
Social and family support for an obese individual's weight-loss program are important. A few words of support can go a long way in the motivation of obese individuals.

Obesity is a serious personal and public health problem in the United States. It has repeatedly been shown that losing weight and maintaining that weight loss are very difficult tasks to accomplish. The recently developed behavior modification approach appears to offer the greatest opportunity for success.

An attack on childhood obesity is extremely important. If your child is overweight, take it seriously and with the help and guidance of your pediatrician develop an appropriate weight-loss program. Obesity in childhood often leads to a lifetime of obesity with its multitude of psychological and physical impairments.

REFERENCES

1. Brownell K: Behavioral treatments for obesity. *Dietetic Currents* 7:13–18, 1980.
2. Woodhouse S: Obesity as a risk factor. *Medical Journal of Australia* (June suppl):11–12, 1976.
3. Woodhouse S: Obesity as a risk factor. *Medical Journal of Australia* (June suppl):11–12, 1976.
4. Society of Actuaries. Build and Blood Pressure Study, 1959.
5. Brownell K: Behavioral treatments for obesity. *Dietetic Currents* 7:13–18, 1980.
6. Brownell K: Behavioral treatments for obesity. *Dietetic Currents* 7:13–18, 1980.
7. Gordon T, et al: Obesity and cardiovascular disease: the Framingham Study. *Clinics in Endocrinology and Metabolism* 5:367–375, 1976.
8. Brownell K: Behavioral treatments for obesity. *Dietetic Currents* 7:13–18, 1980.
9. Brownell K: Behavioral treatments for obesity. *Dietetic Currents* 7:13–18, 1980.
10. Stunkard A, et al: Behavior therapy and self-help programs for obesity, in Munro, JF (ed): *The Treatment of Obesity*. London, MTP Press, 1979, pp. 199–230.
11. Woodhouse S: Obesity as a risk factor. *Medical Journal of Australia* (June suppl) 1:11–12, 1976.
12. Straus R, et al: Operative risks of obesity. *Surgery, Gynecology and Obstetrics*, 116:286–291, 1978.
13. Van Itallie T: Obesity: adverse effects on health and longevity. *American Journal of Clinical Nutrition* 32:2723–2733, 1979.
14. Dyer A, et al: Relationship of relative weight and body mass index to 14 year mortality in the Chicago peoples' Gas Company Study. *Journal of Chronic Diseases* 28:109, 1975.
15. Kannel W, et al: Obesity and cardiovascular disease: the Framingham Study. *Clinics in Endocrinology and Metabolism* 5:367, 1976.
16. Berchtold P, et al: Cardiovascular risk factors and gross obesity. *International Journal of Obesity* 1:219, 1977.
17. Kannel W, et al: Physiological and medical concomitants of obesity: the Framingham Study, in Bray, G. (ed): *Obesity in America*. NIH Publication, no. 79–359, 1979, pp. 125–63.
18. Van Itallie T: Obesity: adverse effects on health and longevity. *American Journal of Clinical Nutrition* 32:2723–2733, 1979.
19. Kannel W, et al: Psyiological and medical concomitants of obesity: the Framingham Study, in Bray G (ed): *Obesity in America*. NIH Publication, no. 79–359, 1979, pp. 125–163.

20. Van Itallie T: Obesity: adverse effects on health and longevity. *American Journal of Clinical Nutrition* 32:2723–2733, 1979.
21. Westlund K, et al: Ten-year mortality and morbidity related to serum cholesterol. *Scandinavian Journal of Clinical Laboratory Investigation* 30 (suppl 127):3, 1972.
22. Chiang B, et al: Overweight and hypertension, a review. *Circulation* 39:403, 1969.
23. Kannel W, et al: Relation of body weight to the development of coronary heart disease. *Circulation* 35: 734, 1967.
24. Keys A, et al: Coronary heart disease: overweight and obesity as risk factors. *Annals of Internal Medicine* 77:15, 1972.
25. Friedman G, et al: The epidemiology of gall bladder disease: observations in the Framingham Study. *Journal of Chronic Diseases* 19:273, 1966.
26. Van Itallie T: Obesity: adverse effects on health and longevity. *American Journal of Clinical Nutrition* 32:2723–2733, 1979.
27. Van Itallie T: Obesity: adverse effects on health and longevity. *American Journal of Clinical Nutrition* 32:2723–2733, 1979.
28. Strauss R, et al: Operative risks of obesity. *Surgery, Gynecology and Obstetrics* 116: 286–291, 1978.
29. Van Itallie T: Obesity: adverse effects on health and longevity. *American Journal of Clinical Nutrition* 32:2723–2733, 1979.
30. Van Itallie T: Obesity: adverse effects on health and longevity. *American Journal of Clinical Nutrition* 32:2723–2733, 1979.
31. Van Itallie T: Obesity: adverse effects on health and longevity. *American Journal of Clinical Nutrition* 32:2723–2733, 1979.
32. Check W, et al: Obesity may reduce survival, increase risk, in breast cancer, *JAMA* 244: 1980.
33. Rimm I, et al: Association between juvenile onset obesity and severe adult obesity in 73,532 women. *American Journal of Public Health* 66:479–481, 1976.
34. Charney E, et al: Childhood antecedents of adult obesity. *New England Journal of Medicine*, 295:6–9, 1976.
35. Wilkinson W, et al: Obesity in childhood: a community study in Newcastle-Upon-Tyne. *Lancet*, February 12, 1977; 350–352.
36. Vulle J, et al: Obesity in 10-year-olds: an epidemiologic study. *Pediatrics* 64:564–567, 1979.
37. Van Itallie T: Obesity: adverse effects on health and longevity. *American Journal of Clinical Nutrition* 32:2723–2733, 1979.
38. Brownell K: Behavioral treatments for obesity. *Dietetic Currents* 7:13–18, 1980.

TEN

Exercise

"Over the past quarter of a century, there has evolved a growing suspicion that the transformation of man by modern technology from a physically active agrarian creature to a sedentary individual one has exacted a toll in ill health."[1]

There has been an increasing awareness among both health professionals and the general population that physical activity may play a significant, and previously largely unexpected, role in the maintenance of our emotional and physical well-being. In recent years, there has been a dramatic rise in the number of Americans who exercise. A 1979 Gallup poll showed that the number of adults who exercise has almost doubled since 1960 and represents nearly 50 percent of our population.[2] Various estimates indicate that the number of joggers now ranges from 10 to 23 million; serious swimmers number approximately 15 million, exercise cyclists, 15 million, and tennis players, 29 million.[3]

The belief that physical activity is beneficial for mind and body is actually not a new thought. Plato is reported to have asked the rhetorical question "And is not bodily habit spoiled by rest and illness, but preserved for a long time by motion and exercise?"[4] Whether or not the beneficial effects of exercise are a "belief" as opposed to medically substantiated fact is a question that has been under intensive recent study by clinicians, epidemiologists, and exercise physiologists.

Much of this research has centered around the problem of heart disease, a natural consequence of the particular importance, in terms of death and disability, that this disease has in our society. The presumed healthful effects of exercise were eagerly anticipated to show some benefit in lessening the risk of developing heart disease. As one author comments, "A therosclerotic cardiovascular disease is now regarded by many as a consequence of faulty life-style that evolves in societies whose populations eat too much of a too rich diet, exercise too little, grow fat, and smoke too much."[5]

EXERCISE AND HEART DISEASE

Exercise is thought by many to be an important element in the reduction of risk from heart attacks. It is believed either to alter the levels of the known major risk factors, such as cholesterol, high blood pressure, smoking, etc, or to exert an independent protective effect. The efficiency of the cardiovascular system is known to be improved by exercise. Several excellent reviews of the available data, examining the relationship of exercise to heart disease risk, have been recently published.[6-9] A closer look at some of these studies will help gain insight and perspective into this relationship.

LEVEL OF WORK ACTIVITY

The concept that the level of physical activity at work was related to the incidence of heart disease probably arose from British social-class data in the early 1950s. These records showed that individuals in professional and business classes were twice as likely to die from heart disease as unskilled workers. In 1953, Morris reported a significant relationship between levels of physical activity and heart disease.[10] The author found that bus conductors, whose job was to walk up and down London's double-decker buses collecting fares, had significant differences in heart disease risk when compared to bus drivers who had little physical activity in their jobs. The conductors experienced only 53 percent of the heart attacks and 46 percent of heart-related deaths as compared to the less active drivers.

The same author compared heart disease in London postmen and a comparable group of more sedentary government clerks.[11] The more active postmen were found to have less heart disease than the physically inactive clerks. A similar study comparing letter carriers and less active postal workers was undertaken in Washington, D.C.[12] The sedentary postal clerks had 1.4 to 1.9 times the risk of heart disease when compared with the physically active letter carriers.

Several reports have been issued from data obtained from San Francisco longshoremen. These men work on the waterfront at various levels of physical activity. Work levels and conditions are well controlled and documented by the longshoremen's union. In a 22-year follow-up study, longshoremen were grouped into high-, medium-, and low-energy expenditure groups.[13] Workers in the high physical activity group had a significantly decreased death rate from heart disease than either the moderate- or low-activity group. The authors concluded that physical activity is protective against fatal heart attacks.

Other studies have been published that demonstrate a protective effect of high levels of physical activity at work. The incidence of heart attacks in a group of North Dakota farmers was found to be only 48 percent of that of nonfarmers.[14] These authors report that in the group of people reporting they performed "some heavy work" there was only an 18 percent incidence of heart disease compared to individuals who claimed they did "no heavy work." In a similar finding among kibbutz workers in Israel, there was reportedly two-thirds less heart disease in the more active workers.[15]

EXERCISE DURING LEISURE TIME

Studies have also focused on the amount of exercise or physical activity spent during leisure time and its relationship to heart disease.

In a recent British study, 17,944 middle-aged male office workers in the civil service were followed for 8.5 years.[16] Men who engaged in vigorous leisure-time exercises or sports had an incidence of heart disease somewhat less than half that of their coworkers who performed no such physical activity. The active group's risk of fatal heart attacks was only about 40 percent that of their sedentary colleagues. Commenting on these findings, the authors state: "The generality of the advantage suggests that vigorous exercise is a natural defense of the body, with a protective effect on the aging heart against ischemia and its consequences."

Harvard alumni were followed for 6 to 10 years for indication of heart disease.[17] Less physically active alumni were found to have a 64 percent greater risk of heart attacks.

Thus, a considerable number of studies have shown a protective effect of physically active occupations and leisure exercise. Sedentary life-styles appear to place individuals at risk for heart disease and, in particular, fatal heart attacks.

The mechanism of this protective action has not been clearly defined. The major question revolved around whether exercise lowers heart risk independently or through modification of the other known risk factors.

Recently published data from the Framingham Study indicate that exercise had an independent effect in lessening cardiovascular risk.[18] In this study, which was skewed because of the sedentary nature of the entire population, there was little correlation between the small amount of exercise reported by these individuals and the major cardiac risk factors.

One proposed protective mechanism of exercise involved the levels of the protective or high density lipoprotein (HDL). HDL has been found in high levels in marathon runners.[19] It has also been demonstrated that levels of HDL increase with physical activity.[20] Finally, HDL levels that are high have been shown to protect against heart disease.[21]

Whatever the exact mechanism, it appears that exercise has a place along with the modification of other known risk factors in programs designed to lessen the risk of heart disease.

EXERCISE AND OBESITY

An active exercise program is now thought to be an important component of any weight-loss program. This has often been neglected in the past because of the belief that the "calorie" benefit of exercise is not significant. It is known, for example, that it takes 1 hour of walking to use up the calories in a slice of cake.[22]

However, the beneficial effect of exercise is not solely in the direct utilization of calories. It is known that exercise actually reduces the appetite in sedentary people.[23] In addition, it increases the metabolic rate for periods up to 48 hours. In this way, your body utilizes more calories than it ordinarily would in the process of daily living.

There are the additional psychological benefits in increased self-esteem and greater self-confidence that are known to be associated with exercise. This is particularly significant in obese individuals who are already victims of guilt and low esteem.

For these reasons, regular exercise should be thought of as a significant and integral part of a comprehensive weight-loss program.

EXERCISE AND CARDIAC REHABILITATION

Approximately 1 million Americans will sustain heart attacks. It has been estimated that there will be 350,000 survivors. The American Heart Association has concluded that one-half of these people will have significant psychological, physiologic, or sociologic disabilities.[24]

Newly developed cardiac rehabilitation exercise programs have become available to help meet this need. There is evidence that these exercise programs can offer some symptomatic and physiologic benefit.[25] Relief of chest pain and improvements in the quality of life are some of the potential benefits of rehabilitation programs. Unfortunately, there is little evidence to support the notion that either the risk of recurrent heart attacks or the ultimate prognosis is altered.

EXERCISE AND YOU

There are many forms and varieties of exercise available to you. Before beginning an exercise program, a physical examination, including an EKG, should be obtained. In certain circumstances, such as age over 40 or the presence of cardiac risk factors, a "stress test" may be obtained. This evaluation prior to beginning active exercise will assure the greatest degree of safety.

Begin your exercise program slowly. As a rule of thumb, do not exercise at a pace that causes such shortness of breath that you cannot carry on a conversation. This is referred to as the "conversational pace" and has been found to correlate well with the heart rate.[26]

The most common form of exercise is jogging. This can be done around a track, but often roads, golf courses, and trails can offer more scenic and less monotonous routes.

Bicycling is a good form of exercise. It is limited in that it requires energy expenditures of varying intensity, pedaling sometimes and coasting others. It is estimated that it takes two to three times longer to get the benefit from bicycling than it does from running or jogging.[27]

Swimming has the obvious disadvantage of requiring a pool and being dependent on weather conditions. Swimming utilizes the smaller muscles of the upper torso and requires approximately twice as long as jogging to get the same benefit.

There are many other physiologically beneficial forms of exercise, including aerobic dance, calisthenics, rope skipping, and stationary running.

We have seen that there are many physical and emotional benefits that can be expected to accrue from a regular exercise program (Tables 10-1 and 10-2. It can offer us many personal benefits, not the least of which is improvement in the overall quality of life.

TABLE 10-1. PHYSICAL BENEFITS OF EXERCISE

Decreased risk of heart disease

Decreased blood pressure

Better weight control

Increased level of conditioning

TABLE 10-2. PSYCHOLOGICAL BENEFITS OF EXERCISE

Increased self-esteem

Greater self-reliance

Decreased anxiety

Improvement in the overall quality of life

REFERENCES

1. Kannel W, et al: Some health benefits of physical activity—the Framingham Study. *Archives of Internal Medicine*, 139:857–861, 1979.
2. Thomas G: Physical activity and health epidemiologic and clinical evidence and policy implications. *Preventive Medicine*, 8:89–103, 1979.
3. Thomas G: Physical activity and health epidemiologic and clinical evidence and policy implications. *Preventive Medicine*, 8:89–103, 1979.
4 Thomas G: Physical activity and health epidemiologic and clinical evidence and policy implications. *Preventive Medicine*, 8:89–103, 1979.
5. Kannel W, et al: Some health benefits of physical activity—the Framingham Study. *Archives of Internal Medicine*, 139:857–861, 1979.
6. Kannel W, et al: Some health benefits of physical activity—the Framingham Study. *Archives of Internal Medicine*, 139:857–861, 1979.
7. Thomas G: Physical activity and health epidemiologic and clinical evidence and policy implications. *Preventive Medicine*, 8:89–103, 1979.
8. Froelicher V, et al: Physical activity and coronary heart disease. *Cardiology*, 65:153–190, 1980.
9. Wyndham C: The role of physical activity in the prevention of ischaemic heart disease. *South African Medical Journal*, 56:7–13, 1979.
10. Morris J, et al: Coronary heart disease and physical activity of work. *Lancet* 2: 1053–1057, 1111–1120, 1953.
11. Morris J: Coronary disease in England. *Cardiology Practice*, 13:85–95, 1962.
12. Kahn H: The relationship of reported coronary heart disease mortality to physical activity of work. *American Journal of Public Health*, 53:1058–1067, 1963.
13. Paffenbarger R, et al: Energy expenditure, cigarette smoking, and blood pressure level as related to death from specific diseases. *American Journal of Epidemiology*, 108:12–18, 1978.
14. Zukel W, et al: Short-term community study of the epidemiology of coronary heart disease. *American Journal of Public Health*, 49:1630–1639, 1959.
15. Brunner D, et al: Myocardial infarction among members of communal settlements in Israel. *Lancet*, December 6, 1980;1207–1210.
16. Morris J, et al: Vigorous exercise in leisure time: protection against coronary heart disease. *Lancet*, December 6, 1980; 1207–1210.
17. Paffenbarger R, et al: Physical activity as an index of heart attack risk in college alumni. *American Journal of Epidemiology*, 108:161–175, 1978.
18. Kannel W, et al: Some health benefits of physical activity—the Framingham Study. *Archives of Internal Medicine*, 139:857–861, 1979.

19. Wood P, et al: Plasma lipoprotein concentrations in middle-aged runners. *Circulation* 50 (suppl 3): 115, 1974.

20. Lopez S, et al: Effect of exercise and physical fitness on serum lipids and lipoproteins. *Atherosclerosis* 20:1–9, 1974.

21. Gordon T, et al: High density lipoprotein as a protective factor against coronary heart disease: the Framingham Study. *American Journal of Medicine* 62: 707–714, 1977.

22. Allen D Weston, et al: The role of physical activity in the control of obesity. *Medical Journal of Australia* 2:434–438, 1977.

23. Allen D Weston, et al: The role of physical activity in the control of obesity. *Medical Journal of Australia* 2:434–438, 1977.

24. Froelicher V, et al: Physical activity and coronary heart disease. *Cardiology* 65:153–190, 1980.

25. Froelicher V, et al: Physical activity and coronary heart disease. *Cardiology* 65:153–190, 1980.

26. Payne F: A practical approach to effective exercise. *AFP* 19:76–81, 1979.

27. Payne F: A practical approach to effective exercise. *AFP* 19:76–81, 1979.

ELEVEN

Stress

"Obviously stress is individually experienced, just as beauty is said to be in the eye of the beholder; this unique experience of stress triggers a constellation of responses peculiar to each individual. Even opposite functions are possible—so, one man's meat is another man's poison."[1]

Over the past few years, it has become increasingly recognized that exposure to stress is a fact of life in contemporary society. Stress and its effects have been popularized in the lay press as well as in the medical and psychiatric literature.

It is becoming more widely accepted that even the stress of ordinary life events can contribute to serious illness and disability. The importance of "life crises" as a factor adversely affecting many people is now established. Stress has been linked to psychosomatic illness, peptic ulcer disease, and heart disease and is known to have a detrimental effect on health and a general sense of well-being.[2]

WHAT IS STRESS?

Despite the popularity and common image of the term "stress," there is actually considerable confusion about its exact meaning. In the lay usage, stress has come to be associated with life events that are thought of as annoying, distressful, or harmful.[3] Terms such as conflict, threat, anxiety, or thrill are often used synonymously.

The perception of and adaptation to events that are "stressful" play a crucial role in determining whether, in fact, they are a negative force on an individual. "Ball players, soldiers, sailors and many others look on stress with such exuberance that their hormonal and neural responses must be different from those of the more sedentary who might look with anxiety or loathing on the same activity."[4]

An early and generally accepted definition of stress by Hans Selye is that it is the nonspecific response of the organism to any demand placed on it.

From an engineering point of view, stress produces strain, and many scientists use the term in the same sense. In this conceptualization, stress is used to describe the individual's response to provoking agents known as stressors. Stressors can be divided into long-term and short-term, depending on the time period over which they act. A more useful division is into environmental and psychological stressors. Environmental stressors would include external factors such as noise, vibration, electric shock, sudden rapid movements, temperature extremes, etc. Psychological or emotional stressors include such things as fear and anxiety.[5]

The confusion in terminology has led to a resultant confusion in many of the studies involving stress. Stress and its relationship to various emotional states has particularly suffered from the lack of precision involved in definition of both of these variables.

In an attempt to ameliorate this problem, the National Conference on Emotional Stress and Heart Disease has offered this contemporary definition of stress: "An obviously painful or adverse force which induces distress or strain upon both the emotional and physical make-up."[6]

It is apparent that stress is highly individual. Whether an event is stressful to someone depends on the individual totality of constitutional factors, including heredity, early growth and development, psychological conditioning throughout life, cultural factors, and morale or group support. It is through this web of interlocking mediating forces that a potential "stressor" must pass. Every individual will thus respond in a unique way to a potentially provoking event. It has been noted that what may be stress producing in some individuals may be enjoyable to others.

STRESS, DEPRESSION, AND PSYCHOSOMATIC ILLNESS

Stress has long been believed to be a risk factor in the development of depression and pychosomatic illness.[7,8] Daily events in life and work in modern Western society often result in a continuous barrage of stressful stimuli. The adjustment to these provocations from both our physical and social surrounding will vary from person to person. The effect a particular event has on the psychological equilibrium of an individual does not necessarily bear an objective relationship to the magnitude of the event. It is the perception of the stressful event that is important. Thus, even seemingly minor daily stress may have a significant impact. "The death of a pet, for example, can be crushing to a lonely, isolated, retired individual with little else in the world."[9]

Significant stressful life events that can lead to either depressive or psychosomatic illness include such things as loss of a loved one, separation, personal defeats, life changes, marital or job dissatisfaction, or onset of a major illness (Table 11-1).[10,11]

Strong empirical evidence that environmental stress can cause psychological and psychosomatic illness has been gleaned from observations of natural and man-made disasters. After a severe tornado hit a rural area in Arkansas, 90 percent of the local residents had acute emotional or psychosomatic after effects.[12] Similarly, a study was done involving 2630 combat-hardened soldiers who had broken down during combat in the Normandy campaign in World War II. It was found that this mental breakdown occurred in previously normal soldiers after about 65 percent of their comrades had become casualties.[13]

The study involving the World War II soldiers with battle fatigue demonstrated an important point. Those soldiers had, for the most part, previously experienced the rigors of combat, often for prolonged periods, with no adverse effects. Upon the loss of 65 percent of their companions, they readily succumbed to the stress of the battlefront.

TABLE 11-1. STRESSFUL LIFE EVENTS THAT CAN LEAD TO DEPRESSION OR PSYCHOSOMATIC ILLNESS

Job dissatisfaction

Lifestyle changes

Family discord

Financial difficulties

Major personal illness

Loss of a loved one

Separation

Defeats (eg, loss of hope, loss of self-esteem)

This clearly shows the significant support that morale and strong social ties can provide against stress.

Happily, these situations are extreme. Yet ordinary events like marriage, loss of a loved one, or job difficulties can induce stress that causes psychopathology. The maladjustment to this stress can sometimes lead to depression or psychosomatic disorders.

Depression is an often unrecognized ailment. Loss of interest in activiy, decreased ability to function, withdrawal, and difficulty sleeping are often seen with this disorder. Depression is an especially serious problem since it can lead to suicide. The magnitude of the problem is apparent when we realize that suicide is the tenth leading cause of death in the United States.

Psychosomatic illness is the expression of psychological distress in the form of bodily symptoms. People undergoing a stressful life situation may develop various physical complaints. The symptomatology in these people is transitory; accordingly, they have been termed "temporary hypochondriacs." There is not necessarily any underlying psychiatric disorder.[14]

Thus, we can see that the stress around us can clearly have an adverse effect on our mental well-being. This is not to say that any stress is necessarily bad. A certain amount of stress is a necessary ingredient to supply the motivation, challenge, and excitement that can make life a more fulfilling experience.

STRESS AND PEPTIC ULCER DISEASE

It is a widely held notion that peptic ulcer disease, or duodenal ulcer, exemplifies the effect of "nerves" on the body. We picture a highly stressed, uptight executive smoking, drinking coffee, and developing an ulcer. While we know that smoking is a risk factor in duodenal ulcer disease, the effect of stress is a separate issue.

Early research at the beginning of this century gave rise to several important concepts.[15]

1. Psychological stimulation was shown to cause secretion of stomach juices (Pavlov).
2. The unconscious could affect bodily functions (Freud).
3. Organic brain lesions could give rise to ulcers (Cushing).
4. Stomach acid secretion was shown to be somehow connected with the development of an ulcer (various authors).

The above data gave fuel to the speculation that psychic stress plays a causative role in the development of duodenal ulcers. Careful scientific scrutiny of this information, however, reveals that, in fact, no cause and effect relationship between psychological stress and the development of ulcers has been proved.

Recently, a panel of experts met to review the available data and to suggest further studies to elucidate the relationship between stress and peptic ulcer disease. Several studies were found that supported the role of stress in the development of ulcers.[16]

Peptic ulcer disease was found to be almost twice as common among air traffic controllers (a high-stress occupation) as compared to second-class airmen.[17]

In another study, peptic ulcer disease was more often found in men in supervisory roles (foremen) than in craftsmen and executives. Presumably, the direct supervision of workers and the responsibility for their work that constitutes a foreman's job are highly stressful.[18]

An attempt to take a more in-depth look at the psychological forces that interact in patients with peptic ulcer disease was noted. A number of everyday situations such as separation, bereavement, dashed hopes of being cared for, and a wife's pregnancy were stated to have special significance to ulcer patients. These situations allegedly signify frustration of that individual's dependency needs.[19]

In another study, preexisting ulcer disease is noted to be exacerbated in a particular psychiatric milieu. This author found that patients who vacillated between "active-seeking" and "passive-yielding" behavior were more prone to develop worsening of their disease.[20]

These studies point to but do not prove the etiologic role of stress in peptic ulcer disease. Much of the previous work concerning this question has suffered both from the difficulties involved in defining stress and in documenting peptic ulcer disease.

Although there is a great body of information that is highly suggestive of a relationship between stress and peptic ulcer disease, the question is still open. It is probably true that stress does play some still undefined role in this disease.

TYPE A AND TYPE B PERSONALITIES

Previously, it was noted that stressful forces are omnipresent in our modern world. The way in which individuals handle this stress—coping patterns—is determined by an amalgam of factors. Influences from growth and development, heredity, social support structures, cultural factors, and a lifetime of conditioning all interact in a particular way in each individual. The way in which an individual interprets and adapts to a stressful situation will determine if it produces strain or "distress" on that person's emotional and physical health.

Recently, there has been a great deal of research on individual stress differences and behavior patterns.[21] Early in the 1960s, Friedman, Rosenman, and Carroll reported a relationship between a particular pattern of behavior and the incidence of heart disease. Further study allowed them to separate individuals into two main patterns of behavior or personality types: type A and type B. They reported that people with type A personality are more prone to heart disease.[22] Indeed, recently published reports tend to confirm the hypothesis that stress in a type A personality is an independent risk factor for heart disease.[23]

The type A personality pattern is characterized by excessive activity, competitiveness, aggressiveness, preoccupation with deadlines, hostility, impatience, time urgency, and abruptness of gesture and speech (Table 11-2). This personality type apparently responds to stressful stimuli with a much greater degree of physiologic arousal than a type B personality.[24]

TABLE 11-2. CHARACTERISTICS OF TYPE A PERSONALITY

Excessive activity

Competitiveness

Aggressiveness

Hostility

Impatience

Time urgency

Preoccupation with deadlines

Abruptness of gesture and speech

The type B behavior pattern is characterized by a relative lack of type A traits. In other words, these individuals display no sense of time urgency, no free-floating hostility, are able to relax without guilt, etc[25] (Table 11-3).

Stressful life situations that are confronted by a person with type A personality lead to more physiologic activity, which in turn leads to a greater incidence of heart and blood vessel disease. It is also likely that an individual with this personality type will more often have the traditional risk factors for heart disease such as smoking and high cholesterol.

TABLE 11-3. CHARACTERISTICS OF TYPE B PERSONALITY

Absence of the features associated with a type A personality

No sense of time urgency

No free-floating hostility

Ability to relax without guilt

It is becoming increasingly apparent that stress and our individual reactions to it can have both emotional and physical sequelae. In the next section, the relationship of stress and heart disease will be more closely examined.

STRESS AND HEART DISEASE

The possible interrelationship between stress, patterns of behavior, and heart disease, although recently popularized, is not a new concept in medicine. In 1892, Sir William Osler, in his description of cardiac patients, declared that they were people who "worked at maximum capacity, incessantly striving for success in commercial, professional or political life."[26] This description is not very different from the classic characterization of an individual with the coronary-prone personality type A.

In recent years, it has become clear that the known cardiac risk factors did not account for many of the heart disease patients who were being seen by physicians. It seemed likely that some other variable was missing. Many have suggested that stress is the "missing link" in the etiology of heart disease.

From a conceptual point of view, a very thought-provoking "explanation" of the role of stress in heart disease has been advanced.[27] In this schema, early man in a primeval setting was confronted with all kinds of threatening situations. Faced with these dangers, he had to physically deal with them, that is, fight or flee. His adrenal glands poured forth adrenaline (catecholamines) that released free fatty acids from body stores to be utilized as fuel for his muscles.

Modern society still bombards us with stressful stimuli, but we no longer can deal with them in a physical way. The adrenaline still flows, and the free fatty acids are still made available, but there is no contracting muscle to utilize this fuel. These fatty-acid and adrenaline surges travel a different path and find their way to the blood vessels supplying the heart.

This schema is neither proof of a relationship between heart disease and stress nor a scientifically documented chain of events. It is fascinating in that it is in fact consistent with much of what is now known.

There have been many reports suggesting a link between stress and heart disease. One report from a hospial in Londonderry, Northern Ireland, has recorded a steady and sometimes steep rise in heart attack victims each year since civil unrest began there.[28]

A Swedish study compared patients with clinical heart disease, patients with risk factors for heart disease, and healthy patients.[29] They found that the risk of developing clinical heart disease in people exposed to psychological stress was six times greater than in controls. Sources of stress that were elicited included work, family life, and education.

Two large prospective studies were recently published investigating the relationship of type A personality and heart disease. These studies have more statistical significance than prior work because of their excellent methodology and prospective design. The Western Collaborative Group Study evaluated the association of type A personality and heart disease in 3154 men, aged 39 to 59 years, followed for 8.5 years.[30] This study showed that men with type A personality had a significantly increased risk for heart disease and that risk was independent of known risk factors.

The Framingham Study followed 1674 men and women for 8 years in an attempt to study a possible link between type A personality and heart disease.[31] The investigators concluded that type A personality is an important and independent risk factor for the development of heart disease in both men and women. The Framingham Study is the first one to demonstrate that women with type A personality were at increased risk for heart disease. The risk in men was only demonstrated in white-collar workers.

There is still some difference of opinion in medical circles concerning the risk of stress and type A personality in the development of heart disease. Recent evidence, especially the newly reported Framingham Study, gives a good deal of credence to the significance of these factors as independent risk factors. It seems reasonable to conclude that stress and personality type A are indeed significant and important risk factors in the development of heart disease.

"Control of individual risk factors has not been strikingly effective in preventing coronary disease, and a substantial reduction in its prevalence seems unlikely without a complete change in our materialistic society which encourages and rewards aggressive, competitive, and stress-producing habits at work and leisure."[32]

STRESS AND SUDDEN DEATH

Sudden death is the death, usually within minutes, of a person not previously considered at risk. Approximately 67 percent of these people die before they can be brought to a hospital.[33]

In the United States, this phenomenon accounts for the loss of 1200 lives daily, or almost one per minute. Among men aged 20 to 64 years, it is the leading cause of death, responsible for 32 percent of fatalities in this age group. It is estimated that almost 25 percent of these victims had no prior symptoms of heart disease.[34]

Sudden death is now believed to result from aberrant electrical activity in the heart. This activity leads to abnormal heart rhythms that in turn compromise the heart's ability to pump effectively. When the electrical activity degenerates heart muscle movements into uncoordinated quavering motions (known as ventricular fibrillation), death rapidly ensues. This is especially tragic since ventricular fibrillation can often be readily reversed in the hospital with no adverse sequelae. It is also apparent that although some of these patients have underlying heart disease, many do not.

Stress has been implicated in the etiology of the sudden death syndrome. Human and animal evidence has shown that psychological stress can lead to abnormal heart rhythms and sudden death.[35-37] Nineteen patients with already established abnormal heart rhythms were given mildly stressful tasks, such as mental arithmetic, to perform. Eleven of these patients developed significant worsening of their heart rhythms.[38]

In a review of 275 cases of sudden death taken from newspaper accounts, eight particular life situations were identified:[39]

1. Twenty-one percent died upon receiving news of the collapse or death of a close person.
2. Nine percent died on the threat of imminent loss of a close person.
3. Twenty percent died during the first three weeks of grief for a loved one.
4. Three percent died during mourning or on the anniversary of the death of a loved one.
5. Six percent died upon loss of self-esteem or public humiliation.
6. Twenty-seven percent died when faced with extreme personal danger or threat of injury.

7. Seven percent died shortly after the danger had passed.
8. Six percent died during an emotional reunion, triumph, or happy ending.

This anecdotal information is interesting because it illustrates the importance of the role of stressful life events in sudden death. The particular situations identified are not representative in that they were taken from newspaper reports. As the author recognizes, it is only a particular subset of episodes of sudden death that will draw the attention of the press.

It seems likely that stress is a factor in the sudden death syndrome. Whether or not there is underlying heart disease, individuals under stress are potentially at risk.

The way in which an individual copes with stress may be an important determinant in its physiologic effects. Certainly, in heart disease, the behavior patterns known as type A seem to be related to adverse effects of stress. In a similar manner, the reduction of stress and learned changes in coping patterns may reduce the risk of sudden death.

STRESS AND OCCUPATION

"Although occupational stress has never been classified a public health problem, it may be one of America's most significant causes of illness."[40]

Most people spend more than half their waking hours at work. Investigators have found that the work environment can be a significant source of stress to an individual. It is thus apparent that if stress is a factor in disease, then occupation and the work environment can affect a worker's well-being.

Stress is perceived and adapted to in an individual manner by different people. It has been noted that personality type A is a coping pattern that is unsuccessful in that it can lead to illness. A study of the distribution of type A and B behavior patterns in the general population revealed that 50 percent of people are classified as type A.[41]

The type A personality with its competitiveness and aggressiveness is often rewarded in today's work environment. Indeed, occupational stress may encourage and promote the development of this personality. People who work as switchboard operators, taxicab drivers, assembly line workers, managers, etc—that is, in jobs that demand speed and that are highly time pressured—may adapt by developing a type A personality.[42]

In a study of 1540 workers in a large financial institution, a significant relationship between occupational stress and disease was found.[43] Interestingly, both overstressed and understressed workers were at higher risk for illness. This is consistent with the theoretical notion that both overstimulation and understimulation are sources of stress in humans.

Several important sources of stress in the work environment have been identified[4] (Table 11-4).

TABLE 11-4. POTENTIAL SOURCES OF STRESS IN THE WORK ENVIRONMENT

Work overload

Relationships at work

Job satisfaction

Job involvement

Responsibility for things and people

Lack of participation in decision making

Overpromotion

Role ambiguity

From Davidson.[25]

Work Overload
A strong association between anxiety and workload in type A people has been noted in several occupations such as university computer operators, accountants, and managers.

Relationships at Work
Type A individuals often are unhappy with the work of subordinates and have poor relations with their supervisors. It has been observed that type A personalities tend to work alone and impose deadlines and increased workloads on themselves. This serves to alienate them, and they lose the buffer that coworker support could offer against stress.

Job Satisfaction

Job dissatisfaction has been shown to be an important source of stress in an individual. There is no difference between type A and B personalities and their reported degree of job satisfaction.

Job Involvement

Intense job involvement associated with competitiveness, aggressiveness, working late, and so on are characteristic of type A personalities. Such involvement can lead to significant stress. Stress in the work environment may potentially contribute to much of the illness that has been discussed. Certainly, it can be a source of anxiety that can interfere with marital and family relations and affect the overall welfare, happiness, and sense of well-being of an individual.

STRESS AND PREVENTION

Stress prevention can be accomplished either by lessening the stressful forces in our life or changing our adaptation to those forces.

The materialistic, aggressive, competitive contagion that has gripped the industrialized nations of the world has caused many of us to lose track of some of the more fundamental and important things in our life. A basic reassessment of priorities would go a long way toward relieving the stresses to which we oftentimes subject ourselves.

There have been behavior modification programs aimed at our adaptation to stress, that is, changing type A to type B personalities. These have met with some success. It has been noted that these changes are not accompanied by a decrease in the quality or quantity of work output. "Type B individuals are just as likely to be ambitious and intelligent as their type A counterparts. Moreover, unlike that in type A individuals, the drive in type Bs is associated with security and confidence rather than irritability and annoyance."[45]

Behavior modification programs utilize such techniques as physical and mental relaxation, group sessions, and work-habit changes like planning fewer meetings, scheduling telephone calls, and setting aside free time periods. Support and encouragement from family and friends are considered important.[46]

It seems unlikely that behavior modification programs will occur on any large scale in the near future. When corporate personnel departments become more aware that these programs result in no loss of productivity, better employee health (and therefore less sick days), and a better office milieu, there may be more of a coordinated effort in this direction.

For now, it seems that prevention is up to you. Think about what really is important in life. Consider what you can do at your job. Change your work habits in a positive way. Remember, one-half of those of you reading this are personality type A.

REFERENCES

1. Eliot R: Stress and cardiovascular disease. *European Journal of Cardiology* 97–104, 1977.
2. Rahe R: 1. Recent life change stress and psychological depression, *Rhode Island Medical Journal* 63: 98–100, 1980.
3. Roscoe A: Stress and workload in pilots. *Aviation, Space, and Environmental Medicine*, April 1978, 630–636.
4. Wolf S: The role of stress in peptic ulcer disease. *Journal of Human Stress*, June 1979, 27–37.
5. Roscoe A: Stress and workload in pilots. *Aviation, Space, and Environmental Medicine*, April 1978, 630–636.
6. Hendrix GH (ed): National Conference on Emotional Stress and Heart Disease. *Journal of the South Carolina Medical Association* 72 (suppl.): 1976.
7. Rahe R: 1. Recent life change stress and psychological depression, *Rhode Island Medical Journal* 63: 98–100, 1980.
8. Barsky A: Patients who amplify bodily sensations. *Annals of Internal Medicine* 91:63–70, 1979.
9. Barsky A: Patients who amplify bodily sensations. *Annals of Internal Medicine* 91:63–70, 1979.
10. Barsky A: Patients who amplify bodily sensations. *Annals of Internal Medicine* 91:63–70, 1979.
11. Rahe R: 1. Recent life change stress and psychological depression, *Rhode Island Medical Journal* 63: 98–100, 1980.
12. Dohrenwend B, et al: Some issues in research on stressful life events. *Journal of Nervous and Mental Disease* 166:7–15, 1978.
13. Dohrenwend B, et al: Some issues in research on stressful life events. *Journal of Nervous and Mental Disease* 166:7–15, 1978.
14. Barsky A: Patients who amplify bodily sensations. *Annals of Internal Medicine* 91:63–70, 1979.
15. Wolf S: The role of stress in peptic ulcer disease. *Journal of Human Stress*, June 1979, 27–37.

16. Wolf S: The role of stress in peptic ulcer disease. *Journal of Human Stress*, June 1979, 27–37.

17. Cobb S, et al: Hypertension, peptic ulcer and diabetes in air traffic controllers. *JAMA* 224: 489–492, 1973.

18. Dunn JP, et al: Frequency of peptic ulcer among executives, craftsmen, and foremen. *Journal of Occupational Medicine* 4: 343–348, 1962.

19. Engel GL: Psychological aspects of gastrointestinal disorders, Reiser MF (ed): *American Handbook of Psychiatry*. New York: Basic Books,, 1975, pp. 653–692.

20. Weisma AD: A study of the psychodynamics of duodenal ulcer exacerbations with special reference to treatment and the problem of specificity. *Psychosomatic Medicine* 18: 2, 1956.

21. Davidson M, et al: Type A coronary-prone behavior in the work environment. *Journal of Occupational Medicine* 22: 375–383, 1980.

22. Friedman M, et al: *Type A Behavior and Your Heart*. London, Wildwood House, 1974.

23. Haynes S, et al: The relationship of psychosocial factors to coronary heart disease in the Framingham Study. *American Journal of Epidemiology* 111:37–58, 1980.

24. Dembroski T, et al: Physiologic reactions to social challenge in persons evidencing the Type A coronary-prone behavior pattern. *Journal of Human Stress* 3: 2–9, 1977.

25. Davidson M, et al: Type A coronary-prone behavior in the work environment. *Journal of Occupational Medicine* 22: 375–383, 1980.

26. Haynes S, et al: The relationship of psychosocial factors to coronary heart disease in the Framingham Study. *American Journal of Epidemiology* 111:37–58, 1980.

27. Clayton M: Risk factor in heart disease. *Medical Journal of Australia* 973–975, 1977.

28. Parkes W: Stress factors in Northern Ireland as seen from a coronary care unit. *Practioner* 218:409–416, 1977.

29. Orth-Gomer K, et al: impact of psychological stress on ischemic heart disease when controlling for conventional risk indicators. *Journal of Human Stress*, March 1980, 7–15.

30. Rosenman RH, et al: Coronary heart disease in the Western Collaborative Group Study: final follow-up experience of 8½ years. *JAMA* 233:872–877, 1975.

31. Haynes S, et al: The relationship of psychosocial factors to coronary heart disease in the Framingham Study. *American Journal of Epidemiology* 111: 37–58, 1980.

32. Bethell H: Stress and C.H.D. *Lancet*, July 10, 1976; 94.

33. Kones R: Emotional stress, plasma catecholamines, cardiac risk factors, and atherosclerosis. 327–336.
34. Lown B: Sudden cardiac death: the major challenge confronting contemporary cardiology. *American Journal of Cardiology* 43: 313–328, 1979.
35. Lown B: Sudden cardiac death: the major challenge confronting contemporary cardiology. *American Journal of Cardiology* 43: 313–328, 1979.
36. Kones R: Emotional stress, plasma catecholamines, cardiac risk factors, and atherosclerosis. 327–336.
37. Engle G: Psychologic stress, vasodepressor (vasovagal) syncope, and sudden death. *Annals of Internal Medicine* 89: 403–412, 1978.
38. Lown B, et al: Roles of psychologic stress and autonomic nervous system changes in provocation of ventricular premature complexes. *American Journal of Cardiology* 41: 979–985, 1978.
39. Engle G: Psychologic stress, vasodepressor (vasovagal) syncope, and sudden death. *Annals of Internal Medicine* 89: 403–412, 1978.
40. Weiman C: A study of occupational stressor and the incidence of disease risk. *Journal of Occupational Medicine* 19: 1977.
41. Davidson M, et al: Type A coronary-prone behavior in the work environment. *Journal of Occupational Medicine* 22: 375–383, 1980.
42. Davidson M, et al: Type A coronary-prone behavior in the work environment. *Journal of Occupational Medicine* 22: 375–383, 1980.
43. Weiman C: A study of occupational stressor and the incidence of disease risk. *Journal of Occupational Medicine* 19: 119–122, 1977.
44. Davidson M, et al: Type A coronary-prone behavior in the work environment. *Journal of Occupational Medicine* 22: 375–383, 1980.
45. Davidson M, et al: Type A coronary-prone behavior in the work environment. *Journal of Occupational Medicine* 22: 375–383,1980.
46. Davidson M, et al: Type A coronary-prone behavior in the work environment. *Journal of Occupational Medicine* 22: 375–383, 1980.

TWELVE

Pollutants, Food Additives, Drugs, and Environmental Factors Associated with the Development of Cancer

The importance of cancer as a cause of death and suffering throughout the world is well known. While other major causes of death in the United States have declined, the cancer death rate has increased to become the second leading cause, responsible for 20 percent of all deaths. Projection of current statistics indicate that by the year 2000 cancer will claim 510,000 lives.[1] From another perspective, the lifetime chance of developing cancer for people born in the United States in 1970 is estimated to be 27.13 percent for men and 27.85 percent for women.[2]

For many years, intensive effort has been directed toward the treatment of cancer with drugs, surgery, radiation therapy, and recently, immunotherapy. Although there have been areas of great success, for example, Hodgkin's disease, acute lymphoblastic leukemia in children, and some other cancer types, for the most part, results have been less than satisfactory.

Much recent information has offered the prospects of a new

concept in the attack on cancer. For the first time, the modification of risk factors and prevention are real possibilities in this devastating disease.

Environmental factors are now believed to be important in the development of most human cancer. It has been estimated that 80 to 90 percent of all cancer is dependent on environmental influences.[3] In the United States, for example, 33 percent of all cancer in men and 10 percent of all cancer in women are directly associated with cigarette smoking.

International cancer incidence rates first became available in the early 1960s. Comparisons of cancer types and rates in parts of the world that differed in personal habits, diet, socioeconomic levels, exposure to drugs, working conditions, and possibly genetic factors gave much support to the role of environmental influences in cancer.[4]

There are many examples of international variations in the types and incidence rates of cancer. Ugandans, Nigerians, and South African blacks are reported to have very low rates of cancer of the voice box (larynx), lungs, stomach, large bowel (colon), rectum, kidney, and brain but are at very high risk for primary liver cancer (a condition that is rare in the United States). Japanese have very low rates for melanoma, Hodgkin's disease, and breast cancer but are at very high risk for stomach cancer.[5]

Further support for the importance of environmental influences comes from the study of migrant populations. For example, when native Japanese moved to California, their offspring experienced a fall in stomach cancer risk and a rise in colon cancer risk that approached the native California Caucasian population.[6]

The concept of environmental influence is used in the broadest possible sense. The effect of drugs, occupational exposure, diet, pollutants, chemical exposure, food additives, and other variables are included in this broad characterization. In this chapter, we will look at these variables. Knowledge of these factors is the first step in prevention.

TOBACCO

Approximately 30 to 35 percent of all cancer deaths among men in the United States are associated with smoking cigarettes. In women, the comparable figure is 5 to 10 percent. As more women smoke, this number is expected to rise. It is projected that within 5 years the lung cancer death rate among women will exceed the rate for breast cancer. Eighty to eighty-five percent of the lung cancer deaths in men and 40 to 45 percent in women are attributable to smoking.[7,8]

Cigarette smoking is associated with the development of cancer of the lung, voice box, throat, feeding tube (esophagus), bladder, and pancreas. This is not to mention the excess death from heart disease and strokes that is elsewhere discussed. Smoking is a major source of entirely preventable death and illness.

ALCOHOL

Alcoholism has been linked to cancer of the mouth, throat, voice box, esophagus, and liver. People who are alcoholics often smoke, and the resultant tumors may be a consequence of the interaction of these factors. It is estimated that 3 to 7 percent of cancer deaths are related to alcoholism. An effect of moderate or small amounts of alcohol intake on the development of cancer has not been demonstrated.

OCCUPATION

Cancer related to occupational exposure has been a recognized problem for many years. Before the turn of the century, it was noted that chimney sweeps, exposed to tar and soot, developed cancer of the scrotum. Since that time, a great deal of information has been accumulated concerning cancer in the work place.

After World War II and with the ever-increasing technological sophistication of our society, a great many new synthetic chemicals have been produced. These newly synthesized chemicals have never before been in contact with man.

The potential risks involved became apparent, and in 1970 the Occupational Safety and Health Act (OSHA) was passed. This has resulted in intensified efforts to control and regulate possible cancer-causing agents in the work environment.

An illustration of the problem can be seen in the case of vinyl chloride. The occurrence of a very rare and fatal type of liver cancer in workers in contact with vinyl chloride strongly suggested an association between this agent and the rare tumor. Unfortunately, in this case, laboratory evidence of the possible cancer-causing nature of this chemical was demonstrated years before but was ignored. It took the development of fatal tumors in humans before action was taken.[9]

There are many other cases of industrial agents causing cancer. For example, benzine may cause leukemia, benzidene may cause bladder cancer, beta naphthylamine may cause bladder cancer, and chloromethyl ether may cause lung cancer (Table 12-1).

Asbestos exposure can greatly increase the risk of lung cancer in cigarette smokers. It is also a cause of the fatal tumor known as mesothelioma, that developed in shipyard workers exposed to asbestos during World War II. A similar increased risk for lung cancer is seen in smokers who work in uranium mines. The interaction between cigarette smoking and exposure to ionizing radiation in this case exacerbates the cancer-producing effect of the smoking.

Occupational dangers also include physical factors. Radiologists are known to be at increased risk of developing cancer, especially leukemia, because of their exposure to ionizing radiation. In a similar way, farmers who have a great deal of exposure to sunlight over many years are at high risk of skin cancer.

The prevention of cancer from occupational exposure is theoretically straightforward. Identify the source of the potential cancer-causing agent and either remove it or prevent worker exposure to it. With the rapid synthesis of new, potentially cancer-causing chemical agents, this is a challenge for the future.

The extent of the problem is difficult to estimate. It has been theorized that occupational exposure is responsible for 20 percent or more of all cancers among men in the United States.[10]

FOOD ADDITIVES

"Mental rejection of food additives is encouraged by reading their names on food labels. Who wants to eat something called sorbitan monostearate? However, who would want to drink a beverage containing trimethylxanthine and chlorogenic acid? (it's coffee)."[11]

There has been a great deal of public and private concern over the safety of food additives. Books in the lay press have appeared extolling the virtues of "natural" foods and condemning "chemical" additives. Food additives have been variously cited as causing illness ranging from cancer to emotional disturbance.

TABLE 12-1. CHEMICALS OR INDUSTRIAL PROCESSES ASSOCIATED WITH INDUCING CANCER IN HUMANS

Chemical or Industrial Process	Main Type of Exposure	Target Organ	Main Route of Exposure
Aflatoxins	Environmental, occupational	Liver	Oral, inhalation
4-Aminobiphenyl	Occupational	Bladder	Inhalation, skin, oral
Arsenic compounds	Occupational, medicinal, and environmental	Skin, lung, liver	Inhalation, skin, oral
Asbestos	Occupational	Lung, pleural cavity, gastro-intestinal tract	Inhalation, oral
Auramine (manufacture of)	Occupational	Bladder	Inhalation, skin, oral
Benzene	Occupational	Bone marrow	Inhalation, skin
Benzidene	Occupational	Bladder	Inhalation, skin, oral
Bis (chloromethyl) ether	Occupational	Lung	Inhalation
Cadmium-using industries	Occupational	Prostate, lung	Inhalation, oral
Chloromethyl methyl ether	Occupational	Lung	Inhalation
Chromium (chromate-producing industries)	Occupational	Lung, nasal cavity	Inhalation
Hematite mining (? radon)	Occupational	Lung	Inhalation
Isopropyl oils	Occupational	Nasal cavity, larynx	Inhalation
Mustard gas	Occupational	Lung, larynx	Inhalation
2-Naphthylamine	Occupational	Bladder	Inhalation, skin, oral
Nickel (nickel refining)	Occupational	Nasal cavity, lung	Inhalation
Soot, tars, and oils	Occupational, environmental	Lung, skin (scrotum)	Inhalation, skin
Vinyl chloride	Occupational	Liver, brain, lungs	Inhalation, skin

The term *food additive* first appeared in federal legislation in 1958.[12] According to the FDA, food additives are: "Substances added directly to food, or substances which may reasonably be expected to become components of food through surface contact with equipment or packaging materials, or even substances that may otherwise affect the food without becoming part of it."

NITRATES, NITRITES, AND NITROSAMINES

Nitrates are commonly found in plants and vegetables. They can be converted by bacteria into compounds known as nitrites. When consumed, nitrites can react in the stomach with so-called secondary amines to form nitrosamines. Nitrosamines are known cancer-inducing compounds. Laboratory animals fed low doses of nitrosamines develop cancer.

For many years, nitrites have been used in the meat-curing process. They are commonly used in the production of red meats such as bologna, ham, weiners, salami, etc.

As noted, when eaten, nitrites can undergo a chemical reaction in the stomach to form the cancer-producing substance nitrosamine. A similar reaction takes place in the process of frying bacon, although in this situation most of the nitrosamines escape into the air. Reductions in the amount of nitrites used in the curing of meats is an appropriate preventive measure.[13,14]

SYNTHETIC ANTIOXIDANTS

Upon exposure to air, foods containing unsaturated fatty acids undergo a reaction and become rancid. Rancid food is not only unappealing, it destroys vitamins A and E and can be injurious. This process readily occurs in meats, ground whole wheat, and unpolished rice.

Antioxidants are compounds such as BHA and BHT (butylated hydroxyanisole and butylated hydroxytolvene), which prevent this process from occurring. In addition to this effect, they are thought to have several other beneficial effects in man.

Laboratory animals fed synthetic antioxidants live longer. This has been associated with the ability of these compounds, similar to the actions of vitamin E, to prevent the formation of so-called free radicals in the body. These compounds are also known to inhibit the cancer-inducing properties of some substances (polycyclic hydrocarbons). In the United States, there has been a recent decline in the incidence of stomach cancer. The addition of BHA and BHT to food is thought to be partly responsible.

Despite all this good news, there has been a good deal of pressure from the public to eliminate these products because they are "chemical food additives." Unfortunately, many large food companies have withdrawn these products from the market.

Another antioxidant used in fruits and potatoes to prevent browning is ascorbic acid.[15]

FOOD COLORING

Early food coloring utilized synthetic dyes made from aromatic compounds. Laboratory evidence indicated that many of these products may be injurious to man. Most of these compounds have since been taken off the market.

Many naturally occurring compounds are now used as food colors. These include: carotene (a precursor of vitamin A), apocarotenal, xanthophyll (found in all green leaves), anthocyanins (found in beets and grapes), caramel ("burnt-sugar coloring"), and ferrous gluconate (added to ripe olives).

MILD INHIBITORS

These products have been used to prevent the formation of mold, especially in bread. Propionate and sorbates are safe and effective in preventing spoilage. They are metabolized in the body to carbon dioxide and water. Certain molds known as aflatoxins grow on corn, soybeans, rice, walnuts, and peanuts and are known to be cancer-inducing agents.

Public pressure against additives has resulted in some bread manufacturers removing these products. There is no sensible reason to discontinue the use of these agents.

ADDITIVES THAT PREVENT BACTERIAL SPOILAGE

The earliest use of food additives was to prevent the bacterial spoilage of food. Vinegar, salt, spices, and the process of smoking were variously used to accomplish this. It is now known that smoke used for this purpose contains cancer-inducing compounds.

Recent agents used to prevent bacterial spoilage include: benzoic acid, esters of parahydroxybenzoates, and sorbic acid. They are all safe and effective.

MONOSODIUM GLUTAMATE

Much has been said about monosodium glutamate. This substance is often added to food to enhance its flavor. Monosodium glutamate is not a chemically synthesized agent. It is the sodium salt of the common amino acid known as glutamic acid. This substance is commonly found in protein, especially plant protein. For example, glutamate comprises 30 percent of the protein in wheat. When monosodium glutamate is ingested, it is utilized in the body as a food.

SACCHARIN

There has been a great deal of public concern about the possible cancer-inducing risk of this nonnutritive sweetener. Another nonnutritive sweetener, cyclamate, was banned from the market in 1970 by the secretary of Health, Education and Welfare because of the findings of a cancer-causing effect in laboratory animals. Because of similar evidence involving saccharin, it was removed from the list of products generally recognized as safe (GRAS) in 1972. In 1977, the FDA proposed an outright ban on saccharin.

In 1978, a large case-control study involving 519 bladder cancer patients and a similar number of controls at various Baltimore hospitals was reported. These investigators found no difference in saccharin or cyclamate intake in either patients or controls. They concluded that they could find no relationship between the use of nonnutritive sweeteners and bladder cancer.[16]

In a 700-page report issued by the director of the FDA's National Center for Toxicology Research, the conclusion was reached that the benefit of saccharin outweighed its risks.[17] By way of illustration, that report makes some startling comparisons. The author, Morris N. Cranmer, asserts that the equivalent sweet dose of sucrose (table sugar) carries 375 times the risk of cancer in laboratory animals of a 12 oz diet soda. He also notes that a typical steak has approximately 20 times the bladder cancer potentiating effect (if extrapolated from rat data) of a can of soda. Similarly, five salted peanuts equal the risk of a can of diet soda.

These comparisons should not be interpreted to imply that steak, peanuts, or sugar are dangerous. They are mentioned in the report to underline the difficulty in interpreting laboratory animal findings in the context of human usage. As Cranmer states, they serve to illustrate our "current inability to extrapolate from high to low doses of chemical additives, as when massive quantities fed to small groups of animals are compared with low-level doses in millions of humans over many years." The report continues. "It is difficult to quantify risk, but if it were possible the lifetime risk from regular use of saccharin or other food additives shown to be marginally carcinogenic (cancer-inducing) might prove less significant than that from consumption of a single pack of cigarettes."

Food additives have come under a great deal of public attack. Food additives do not comprise a single class of compounds acting in a similar way. Rather, they all function in different ways and are quite unique in their risk versus benefit potential. Currently, utilized food additives are generally safe and important agents. Public prejudice against any "additives" have caused many useful products, most of which are clearly beneficial, to be withdrawn by the manufacturers. It should be remembered that there are many "natural" foods that are quite dangerous to your health.

"The most injurious of all 'food additives' is the additional food that is eaten after caloric needs have been satisfied. Overconsumption of food leads to obesity, which is a far greater danger to health than any of the food additives whose safety is now being questioned."[18]

DRUGS AND CANCER

Drugs are of necessity substances that are biologically active. That is, they exert an effect on the physiology and biochemical processes of the body. All drugs undergo an exhaustive procedure of animal testing and extensive human clinical trials before they are released for marketing by the FDA. This procedure allows for the detection of possible side effects or dangers associated with the use of the drug.

However, the detection of possible cancer-inducing properties of a drug is not as straightforward. Testing with bacterial systems, insect systems, and laboratory animals have all been utilized. There can be a long lag period between the administration of a cancer-inducing agent and the clinical appearance of a tumor. Therefore, any association between a drug and the development of cancer is often difficult to identify or substantiate.

An extensive review of the link between drugs and cancer has just

TABLE 12-2. DRUGS ASSOCIATED WITH INDUCING CANCER IN HUMANS

Drug	Cancer Type
Radioactive drugs (phosphorous P^{32}, radium, mesothorium, thorotrast)	Organs where concentrated (Acute leukemia, osteosarcoma, nasal sinus carcinoma, angiosarcoma of the liver)
Chlornaphazine	Bladder cancer
Arsenic	Skin cancer
Methoxy psoralen	Skin cancer
Phenacetin-containing drugs	Renal cell carcinoma bladder cancer (?)
Alkylating agents (melphalan, cyclophosphamide, chlorambucil, dihydroxy, bulsulfan, and others)	Acute nonlympholytic leukemia, bladder, other sites (?)
Immunosuppressive agents (azothioprine)	Lymphoma, skin cancer, soft-tissue sarcoma, melanoma(?), liver and gallbladder(?), lung cancer(?)
Androgen-anabolic steroids	Liver cancer (hepatocellular carcinoma)
Estrogen-containing drugs: Prenatal (DES); Postnatal (DES, conjugated estrogens, sequential oral contraceptives)	Vaginal cancer, endometrial cancer, breast cancer (?), cervical cancer (?), ovarian cancer (?), chloriocarcinoma (?), melanoma (?), liver tumors, benign

Adapted from Hoover.[19]

been completed and published.[19] Much of the following information is taken from that review. There are several drugs that have been clearly established as being capable of inducing cancer in humans (Table 12-2). Although some of these drugs have been withdrawn from the market, several are still used in certain circumstances.

Radioisotopes

Radioisotopes induce cancer through the release of ionizing radiation. Ionizing radiation is a well-established cancer-inducing agent in man. Radioactive phosphorus, which is used in a bone marrow disease called polycythemia vera, has been shown to cause leukemia. Radioiodine used in high doses in the treatment of thyroid cancer is thought to probably increase the risk of leukemia.

Chlornaphazine

This product was taken off the market in 1964. It was used in high doses to treat polycythemia vera and Hodgkin's disease where it was found to cause bladder cancer. Chemically, it is related to B-naphthylamine, which is an agent known to cause bladder cancer in chemical workers.

Inorganic Arsenicals

These agents can cause a peculiar variety of multiple skin cancers when taken internally by man. In lab animals, they demonstrate no such cancer-inducing property.

Methoxypsoralen

This substance is used together with ultraviolet light in the treatment of psoriasis. This treatment is associated with the increased risk of skin cancer.

Phenacetin

This drug is found in various analgesic combinations. When used in high doses, it can cause chronic kidney infections and a particular type of kidney cancer. There may be an association with bladder cancer.

Alkylating Drugs

These drugs are used in the treatment of cancer. They include such agents as melphalan, cyclophosphamide, chlorambucil, and others.

Recently, they have been associated with the development of leukemia after a lag time. In most situations in which they are currently used, the benefits outweigh the risks entailed. However, caution should be advised in using these agents for conditions in which there is an expected long-term survival. In one study, patients who survived 10 years of treatment with these agents had a 12 to 20 percent rate of leukemia.

Immunosuppressive Agents
These agents, such as azothioprine, have been used in organ transplant cases to prevent host rejection of the transplant. Kidney transplant patients given this agent had a 32 percent increase in the risk of lymphoma, and increases in risk for liver cancer, gallbladder cancer, bladder cancer, lung cancer, leukemia, and melanoma have also been reported.

Androgenic-Anabolic Steroids
These agents, such as oxymetholone or methyltestosterone, have been associated with liver cancer. They have been used in certain types of anemia and other conditions.

Diethylstilbestrol (DES)
In 1971, reports of a rare type of vaginal cancer were published in females aged 14 to 22 years. Investigations revealed that their mothers had received the drug diethylstilbestrol (DES) during pregnancy. Thus far, there are 350 such cases reported.

In daughters exposed in utero to this agent, the rate of development of vaginal cancer is between 1 in 1000 to 1 in 10,000. The rate rises very rapidly at age 14, peaks at 19, and then falls off abruptly.

Estrogens and Menopause
Studies now clearly show that so-called estrogen replacement therapy during menopause is related to the development of both cancer of the endometrium and breast cancer. The widespread utilization of estrogens in 1960 in menopausal women was followed by a sharp rise in the incidence of cancer of the endometrium. With the recent decline in use of these agents, there has been a corresponding decrease in the rate of endometrial cancer.

Oral Contraceptives

Endometrial cancer is the only tumor that has been clearly linked to the use of oral contraceptives. In this case, the association is with one type of oral contraceptive and perhaps only one brand, Oracon. This association was noted in users of sequential contraceptives. In particular, the brand Oracon had a sevenfold increase in risk. Sequential oral contraceptives involve the use of estrogen-containing pills during the first half of the menstrual cycle followed by a progestin in the latter half.

In this way, sequential and contraceptives expose the women to the effects of so-called unopposed estrogens, that is, estrogen without concomitant exposure to progestins. This simulates the situation in which estrogens were given to menopausal women who later developed endometrial cancer. Oracon used unopposed estrogens for 2 days longer in the cycle and had a stronger estrogen and weaker progestin than the other brands of sequential pills.

Combination oral contraceptives contain a mixture of both estrogens and progestins in one pill. Some evidence suggests that this type of pill may be associated with a decreased risk of endometrial cancer.

DRUGS SUSPECTED OF CAUSING CANCER

Many drugs have been suspected as possibly inducing cancer in humans (Table 12-3). In these drugs, there is too inconsistent, inconclusive, or inadequate information to draw a firm conclusion.

Chloramphenicol and Phenylbutazone

Both of these drugs have been implicated in case reports as being linked to leukemia. There is no definitive evidence to support this.

Iron Dextran

This injectable iron form is used to correct various anemias. There are reports of a type of cancer known as sarcoma developing at the site of injection of these agents. They have also induced sarcomas in laboratory animals. However, the risk in humans is considered either nonexistent or extremely small.

TABLE 12-3. DRUGS THAT ARE POSSIBLY CANCER PRODUCING IN
HUMANS

Drug	Cancer Type
Chloramphenicol	Leukemia
Iron dextran	Soft-tissue sarcoma (site of injection)
Dilatin	Lymphoma
Phenobarbital	Brain tumors; liver cancer
Amphetamines	Lymphoma
Reserpine	Breast cancer
Progesterone (Depo-Provera)	Cervical cancer
Phenylbutazone	Leukemia
Crude tar ointment	Skin cancer
Clofibrate	Gastrointestinal and lung cancer

Adapted from Hoover.[19]

Diphenylhydantoin (Dilantin)

This drug is commonly used in seizure disorders (epilepsy) and is
known to occasionally produce an increase in lymph gland tissue.
Rarely has the development of cancerous lymph tissue known as
malignant lymphoma been reported. The risk is reportedly minimal.

Phenobarbital

This sedative has been reported to be associated with an increased
incidence of brain and liver tumors. The association has been largely
dismissed. However, further evaluation is needed.

Amphetamines

Amphetamines are sometimes used for weight reduction. There are
reports of an association between amphetamine use and the occurrence
of Hodgkin's disease. Other studies show no such association.

Reserpine

This drug is widely used for the treatment of high blood pressure. Early
reports of a link between reserpine and breast cancer have not been

confirmed. The available evidence indicates that there is no association between breast cancer risk and resperine usage.

Depo-Provera
This injectable progesterone has been reported to be linked to cervical cancer. Further evaluation is necessary before any conclusion can be drawn.

Crude Tar Ointments
These substances contain the known cancer-inducing agents known as polycylic hydrocarbons. They are used in the treatment of psoriasis. A recent study indicates that they may increase the risk of skin cancer.

Clofibrate
This drug has been reported to increase the risk of gastrointestinal cancers. The association was noted during studies to evaluate clofibrate's ability to lessen the risks of heart disease. The association is not considered definitive because of the small number of patients involved.

Thus, we have seen the magnitude and complexity of the issues concerning the use of drugs and the development of cancer. While the FDA, drug manufacturers, and independent investigators are doing all they can to elucidate these relationships, perhaps the best advice to you and your physician is contained in this axiom:

> There is a time-honored recommendation given to prescribing or consuming drugs, which should lead to the prevention of side effects or late effects, including cancer. That is, any drug should only be used when necessary, and then at the lowest dose and for the shortest period of time required to achieve the desired results.[20]

WATER CONTAMINANTS AND CANCER

The possible role of water contamination in the development of cancer has been an issue of some recent concern. It has been found that in the water treatment process some organic pollutants are not removed from the water. Although harmless in themselves, these compounds are converted to substances such as chloroform upon chlorination of the water. Chloroform has been shown to cause cancer in laboratory animals.

There is some reason to be concerned that the presence of some organic pollutants in water may play a role in inducing cancer in those consuming such water. There have been proposals that cities with populations greater than 75,000 having such organic substances in the water supply utilize further purification techniques. The use of charcoal filters would effectively remove these organic precursors to chloroform.[21]

SOLAR RADIATION AND CANCER

It has been shown that chronic, cumulative radiation from the sun, especially in the ultraviolet frequency 290 to 320 nm, is a causative factor in skin cancer. This can be observed in farmers who often develop multiple skin cancers in exposed portions of the body such as the face and hands.[22]

Another type of skin cancer known as melanoma occurs often on the trunk and extremities. This tumor seems to be associated with intermittent intense exposure to the sun, as might occur during vacations.[23] Melanoma incidence has also been reported to be associated with the occurrence of sunspot activity.[24] During these periods, there is interference with the protective stratospheric ozone layer of our atmosphere.

Skin pigmentation and protective coverings or clothing are known to reduce the risk from these solar-radiation-induced skin cancers.

AIR POLLUTION AND CANCER

The possible relationship between urban air pollution and cancer has been an undecided issue for many years. It is known that lung cancer incidence is higher in urban areas than in rural ones. This holds true after correction for cigarette smoking (the major causative factor in lung cancer). A recent review of the data has led a group of experts to conclude that among male cigarette smokers an additional 10 percent of the cases of lung cancer can be attributed to urban air pollution.[25]

It is apparent that there are a great many influences from our environment that can contribute to the development of cancer. Many of these risk factors are in our control, while others are not.

Certainly, cigarette smoking is a major cause of cancer that we can entirely prevent. Another important step we can take is a change in diet to one low in fat and high in fiber and the avoidance of obesity. The prevention of cancer will take a major personal, governmental, and private-enterprise effort. The optimistic note is that there are a great many significant risk factors that can be eliminated, and the goal of prevention may be more than just a dream.

REFERENCES

1. Schottenfeld D: The epidemiology of cancer: an overview. *Cancer* 47:1095–1108, 1981.
2. Schottenfeld D: The epidemiology of cancer: an overview. *Cancer* 47:1095–1108, 1981.
3. Greenwald P: Cancer and the environment. *Current Concepts in Oncology* 3: 1981.
4. Schottenfeld D: The epidemiology of cancer: an overview. *Cancer* 47:1095–1108, 1981.
5. Schottenfeld D: The epidemiology of cancer: an overview. *Cancer* 47:1095–1108, 1981.
6. Greenwald P: Cancer and the environment. *Current Concepts in Oncology* 3: 1981.
7. Greenwald P: Cancer and the environment. *Current Concepts in Oncology* 3: 1981.
8. Schottenfeld D: The epidemiology of cancer: an overview. *Cancer* 47:1095–1108, 1981.
9. Nelson N: Cancer prevention: environmental, industrial and occupational factors. *Cancer* 47:1065–1070, 1981.
10. Nelson N: Cancer prevention: environmental, industrial and occupational factors. *Cancer* 47:1065–1070, 1981.
11. Jukes T: Current concepts in nutrition, food additives. *New England Journal of Medicine* 297:427–430, 1977.
12. Jukes T: Current concepts in nutrition, food additives. *New England Journal of Medicine* 297:427–430, 1977.
13. Jukes T: Current concepts in nutrition, food additives. *New England Journal of Medicine* 297:427–430, 1977.
14. Nelson N: Cancer prevention: environmental, industrial and occupational factors. *Cancer* 47:1065–1070, 1981.
15. Jukes T: Current concepts in nutrition, food additives. *New England Journal of Medicine* 297:427–430, 1977.
16. Kessler I, et al: Saccharin, cyclamate, and human bladder cancer. No evidence of association. *JAMA*, 240:349–355, 1978.

17. Research Study Calls Sugar Riskier than Saccharin, *Chemical Week,* August 16, 1978: 32–33.
18. Jukes T: Current concepts in nutrition, food additives. *New England Journal of Medicine* 297:427–430, 1977.
19. Hoover R, et al: Drug-induced cancer. *Cancer* 47:1070–1080, 1980.
20. Hoover R, et al: Drug-induced cancer. *Cancer* 47:1070–1080, 1980.
21. Nelson N: Cancer prevention: environmental, industrial and occupational factors. *Cancer* 47:1065–1070, 1981.
22. Schottenfeld D: The epidemiology of cancer: an overview. *Cancer* 47:1095–1108, 1981.
23. Schottenfeld D: The epidemiology of cancer: an overview. *Cancer* 47:1095–1108, 1981.
24. Houghton A, et al: Increased incidence of malignant melanoma after peaks of sunspot activity. *Lancet,* April 8, 1978; 759–60.
25. Nelson N: Cancer Prevention: Environmental, Industrial and Occupational Factors. American Cancer Society, 1981.

THIRTEEN

Alcohol

Alcohol abuse is known to be associated with serious illness and suffering, severe psychological and social maladjustment, family and marital discord, loss of productivity, violent crimes, automobile accidents and deaths, suicide, a decrease in life expectancy of 8 to 12 years, and even mental and physical impairment in the unborn children of known alcoholic mothers. Yet it is widely known that some 9 million people in the United States abuse alcohol.[1]

Alcohol has a well-accepted place in our society and culture. It is traditionally used to celebrate happy occasions, weddings, anniversaries, and the like. Certainly, a little "Christmas cheer" cannot be thought of as harmful. However, we are surrounded by media advertising that not only romanticizes alcoholic beverages but supports the notion that heavy drinking is "sexy" and "macho." Since the days of Prohibition and perhaps even before, alcohol has become part of our heritage, with tales of speakeasies, bathtub gin, and Eliot Ness.

Alcohol is a potent and dangerous drug to which millions of

people have regular and free access on a daily basis. It is so accepted in our society that most would be shocked to learn they are taking a drug.

Illustrative of the problem is this comment by David Archibald, executive director of the Addiction Research Foundation of Ontario:[2]

Three years ago when we reported that almost 20% of our high school students had tried marijuana, parents and school officials reached the edge of panic. A few months ago when we reported that almost 80% of high school students drank alcohol, and many of them were drinking frequently, there was one collective yawn. Even worse, there was a feeling of relief that at last youngsters in our school had come to their senses and had come back to something we could all accept.

Ten percent of the population that imbibes alcohol become alcohol abusers. What is meant by this term is the development of physical or psychological dependence on alcohol to cope with daily life events such as family problems, work stress, financial difficulties, and a variety of other problems. When this dependence grows to the point of causing problems in daily living, that individual is generally considered an alcoholic.

The National Council on Alcoholism has defined alcoholism "as a chronic, progressive and potentially fatal disease. It is characterized by tolerance and physical dependency or pathologic organ changes or both—all the direct or indirect consequences of the alcohol ingested."[3] In this definition, tolerance refers to the fact that an alcoholic needs greater quantities of alcohol to get effects equal to those obtained with lesser amounts before. Physical dependency is considered present when an individual experiences physical signs and symptoms upon either drinking less or stopping the consumption of alcohol.

We have noted that one out of ten people exposed to alcohol will become alcohol abusers or alcoholics. It is reasonable to consider what it is that distinguishes a social drinker from a problem drinker. There are several "warning signs" that indicate a social alcohol consumer may be crossing the line to become an alcoholic (Table 13-1).

ALCOHOL-CONTAINING BEVERAGES

A closer look at the process by which various alcoholic beverages are produced will serve as the basis for consideration of the problems associated with alcohol.

TABLE 13-1. WARNING SIGNS THAT MAY
INDICATE AN ALCOHOL ABUSER IS BECOMING
AN ALCOHOLIC

Excessive drinking in normal situations

Drinking alone

Drinking to reduce anxiety, apprehension, or anger

Drinking used to help fall asleep

Early-morning drinking

Loss of memory and blackouts

Yeasts are common microscopic organisms that break down natural vegetable sugars as a source of energy. The action of the yeast on the sugars is mediated through enzymes in the process known as fermentation. Fermentation produces energy for the yeast and yields alcohol as a by-product of the reaction.

The particular variety of alcoholic beverages thus produced will depend on the source of the natural sugar. Thus, wine is the product of the fermentation of fruit juices, beer from malted grains, and mead from honey. As the concentration of alcohol increases, the yeasts lose their ability to continue this process. Fermentation ceases when the concentration of alcohol reaches 14 percent.

Alcoholic beverages that contain higher concentrations of alcohol are produced by the process of distillation. The fermented product is heated so that the alcohol, which has a lower boiling point than water, is evaporated off. This evaporated alcohol is condensed and collected in a series of coils. This process results in a concentration of alcohol that is higher than that in the original product of fermentation.

The many varied distillates that can be thus produced depend on the particular fermentation product used. For example, brandy is distilled from wine, and whiskey is distilled from malted grains. Many alcoholic beverages also contain flavorings, or they can be a mixture of various distillates and are then known as blended.

It is apparent that the concentration of alcohol in any given alcoholic beverage is highly variable. This concentration is usually expressed as the percentage of alcohol per unit volume. Beer has the lowest alcohol concentration, approximately 5 percent; wines vary from 9 to 12.5, and hard liquor can be 40 percent or higher. The greater the alcohol concentration of a beverage, the more alcohol or intoxifying effect it exhibits per unit of volume consumed. For example, 12 oz of beer has the same amount of alcohol as 5 oz of wine, 3 oz of sherry or port, or 1.5 oz of whiskey.[4]

Another way to express the concentration of alcohol involves the use of the term "proof." Proof is numerically twice the alcohol concentration; thus, 80 proof whiskey is 40 percent alcohol.

PROBLEMS OF ALCOHOL ABUSE

Social Problems

There are many ways to look at the adverse social consequences associated with alcohol abuse. Its manifold effects range from disruption of family life to psychiatric hospital admissions to exposure to violent personal injury or death. Finally, alcohol abuse imposes a huge burden on our national coffers. It has been estimated that in 1971 the cost in health-care dollars was $31.4 billion. Ten percent of all health-care expenditures in the United States are a result of alcohol abuse and the various illness associated with it.[6]

Violent Criminal Activity

A Canadian inquiry into drug use and its effects found: "Of all drugs used medically or non-medically, alcohol has the strongest and most consistent relationship to *crime*."[7] They found that alcohol is highly associated with crimes against persons, including sex crimes. A review of Canadian prison statistics found that serious drinking problems were found in those convicted of 33 percent of murders, 38 percent of attempted murders, 54 percent of manslaughters, 39 percent of rapes, 42 percent of other sexual offenses, and 61 percent of assaults.

An epidemiologic review of causes of death in alcoholics further substantiated this tendency toward violence. Approximately 20 percent of alcoholics died from violent causes, including homicide, suicide, and accidents.[8]

Auto Accidents

Alcohol consumption is causally related to 50 percent of highway fatalities, 25,000 deaths, and 800,000 accidents per year.[9,10] From another perspective, alcohol has been linked to 30 percent of highway accidents, 22 percent of home accidents, and 16 percent of occupational accidents.

Industry

Alcoholic workers are reported to be absent from work 2.5 times more frequently than nonalcoholics.[11] Besides the days lost from work, the general level of employee competence is impaired with increased numbers of on-the-job accidents.

Psychiatric Hospitalizations

Admissions to various psychiatric facilities for alcohol-related problems range from 10 to 50 percent of all admissions. The more long-term state mental hospitals report that fully one-half of their male admissions between the ages of 35 and 64 are alcohol associated.[12]

Social Service

Social service agencies indicate that almost one-half of their case loads deal with problems related to alcohol. These include a broad range of personal and family problems that are caused or exacerbated by alcohol. Marriage failures, divorce, job difficulties, and legal problems are all commonly noted. Perhaps the most tragic consequence is the so-called "battered child syndrome" in which alcohol plays a notorious role.[13]

ALCOHOL AND HEALTH

It is well known that too much alcohol is bad for your health. Alcoholics suffer from a wide range of chronic disabling and often fatal diseases that are clearly related to their alcohol consumption (Table 13-2). They are also prone to other illness because of their generally vulnerable physical condition and lack of resistance.

In general, there has been a lack of concise information about the relative prevalence of the various alcohol-related diseases. A recent review of the available data revealed some interesting findings.[14]

Several studies demonstrated that alcoholics had a surprisingly high rate of heart disease, varying from 20 to 59 percent. Cirrhosis of the liver (a disease characterized by progressive injury and scarring of

TABLE 13-2. MEDICAL PROBLEMS COMMONLY FOUND IN ALCOHOLICS

Organ or System	Manifestation
Blood-forming elements	Anemia
Liver	Fatty liver, alcoholic hepatitis, cirrhosis
Pancreas	Pancreatitis
Gastrointestinal	Esophagitis, gastritis, peptic ulcer, bleeding esophageal varices, diarrhea
Cardial	Cardiomyopathy (injury to heart muscle), cardiomegaly (enlarged heart), congestive heart failure
Muscle	Muscle weakness
Nervous system	Withdrawal symptoms, tremors, hallucinations, seizures, delirium tremens (DTs), peripheral neuropathy
Nutritional disorders	Niacin deficiency, thiamine deficiency, riboflavin deficiency, pyridoxine deficiency, folic acid deficiency, vitamin C deficiency

Adapted from Alcoholism—Medical Consequences of Therapy, U.S. Pharmacist, June/July 1980.

the liver) was seen in only 5 percent of all alcoholics, while peptic ulcers and gastritis were seen in 10 percent. Chronic lung disease (which is causally linked to the heavy-smoking characteristic of most alcoholics) was found in from 10 to 25 percent of people. Finally, a type of nerve damage known as peripheral neuropathy was found in another 2 to 20 percent.

Alcoholics were found to have a decreased life expectancy of from 8 to 12 years. Their death rates were two to three times the expected norms. Cirrhosis was the cause of death in from 5 to 15 percent. Another 20 percent died of violent causes such as homicide, suicide, and accidents. However, the major cause of death was heart disease, which accounted for 30 to 50 percent of all deaths. The heart disease rate was twice that expected.

ALCOHOL AND HEART DISEASE

There are actually three different types of heart disease specifically associated with alcohol.[15]

So-called alcoholic cardiomyopathy is responsible for 75 to 80 percent of the heart disease linked to alcohol. This is direct damage to and destruction of the heart muscle fibers by a toxic effect of alcohol. Scarring can result in a loss of heart-pumping capabilities.

An additional 10 to 15 percent of patients will have heart failure due to nutritional or beriberi heart disease. This is a result of a vitamin B_1 (thiamine) deficiency that is seen in alcoholism as a result of disturbances in the electrical conducting system of the heart. This is the system that controls the rate and rhythm of heart contraction. The disturbances are thought secondary to a low blood serum potassium and magnesium.

ALCOHOL METABOLISM

It is important to look at the metabolism of alcohol—in other words, how alcohol is handled by the body and eventually made harmless or detoxified. Previously, we mentioned that alcoholics exhibited tolerance. That is, they seemed to be able to handle more alcohol at a faster rate than nonalcoholics. This is a concept that must be explained in any discussion of the metabolism of alcohol.

There are several organ systems that are known to eliminate drugs from the body. These include the lungs, kidney, liver, skin, and gastrointestinal tract. Alcohol is metabolized by the liver. The breakdown of alcohol into harmless degradation products is accomplished with the aid of an enzyme known as alcohol dehydrogenase.

There is a second postulated mechanism in the liver that is thought to detoxify alcohol. This system is known as the "microsomal ethanol oxidizing system." Its importance is that it is believed that chronic alcoholics who ingest alcohol have the capability of enhancing or "inducing" this system. The result is that they are able to metabolize more alcohol at a faster rate. This theory would help explain tolerance on a biochemical level. It is also considered a possibility that the detoxification process involving alcohol dehydrogenase is also accomplished more readily in alcoholics.

Information about these biochemical steps has made possible predictions about the rate of alcohol metabolism in the intoxicated person. The most accepted rate of clearance of alcohol from the blood is 20 mg %/hr in the alcoholic.[16] For example, in a nonalcoholic, it would take 10 hours to reduce an alcohol blood level from 200 mg % to zero. Chronic alcoholics can metabolize blood alcohol at a more rapid rate. It has been shown that a rate of 10 mg %/hr is a reasonable estimate. Thus, in the same 10-hour period, a chronic alcoholic could clear an alcohol blood level of 300 mg % to zero.

It has been approximated that an average 150-lb man could metabolize two-thirds to 1 oz of 90-proof liquor or 8 to 12 oz of beer an hour. The popular notion that drinking coffee after alcohol consumption will help sober you up is a misconception. However, it is true that eating food will slow down the rate of entry of alcohol into the blood stream.

Serum blood levels of alcohol are directly related to the degree of functional impairment (Table 13-3). The serum blood level, in turn, is dependent on the amount you drink, the period of time over which you drink it, and your rate of metabolism. The higher the serum blood level, the more "drunk" you are.

ALCOHOL AND HEREDITY

It is common to think of most, if not all, psychiatric disorders as stemming from environmental rather than genetic factors. Certainly, alcoholism would seem to fit into that category. It is known, for example, that alcoholism "runs" in families. It superficially appears to be learned behavior. In a sense, it is a maladjusted familial coping pattern; 25 percent of the brothers or fathers of alcoholics are themselves alcoholic.[17]

Recent studies reveal the rather surprising result that this is not true at all. Alcoholism has been clearly shown to have a genetic, inherited component. Furthermore, the influence on males of being raised in an alcoholic family does not appear significant. In other words, environmental factors played no measurable role, while genetic ones did.

TABLE 13-3. EFFECTS OF INCREASED BLOOD ALCOHOL LEVEL

Blood Alcohol Level (%)	Average Effects
.02	Reached after approximately one drink; light or moderate drinkers feel some effect, eg, warmth and relaxation.
.04	Most people feel relaxed, talkative, and happy. Skin may flush.
.05	First sizable changes begin to occur—light-headedness, giddiness, lowered inhibitions, and less control of thoughts may be experienced. Both restraint and judgment are lowered; coordination may be slightly altered.
.06	Judgment somewhat impaired; normal ability to make a rational decision about personal capabilities is affected, eg, concerning driving ability.
.08	Definite impairment of muscle coordination and a slower reaction time; driving ability suspect. Sensory feelings of numbness of the cheeks and lips. Hands, arms, and legs may tingle and then feel numb (legally impaired in Canada and the United States).
.10	Clumsy: speech may become fuzzy. Clear deterioration of reaction time and muscle control (legally drunk in most states).
.15	Definite impairment of balance and movement. The equivalent of a half pint of whiskey is in the blood stream.
.20	Motor and emotional control centers measurably affected; slurred speech, staggering, loss of balance, and double vision can all be present.
.30	Lack of understanding of what is seen or heard; individual is confused or stuporous. Consciousness may be lost at this level, ie, individual passes out.
.40	Usually unconscious; skin clammy.
.45	Respiration slows and can stop altogether.
.50	Death can result.

Adapted from Poley W. et al: Alcoholism: A Treatment Manual, Gardner Press, Inc., 1979, N.Y.

The largest study to demonstrate this was a collaborative American-Danish trial.[18] Children of alcoholic parents who were adopted soon after birth were compared to children of nonalcoholic parents similarly adopted. In this way, the effect of environment (being raised by the alcoholic parent) could be eliminated, leaving only genetic factors. It was found that the children of alcoholics developed alcoholism 3.5 times more frequently than the control population. This clearly showed an effect of genetics, independent of environment, in the development of this disease.

These adopted children of alcoholics were then compared to their nonadopted brothers. The nonadopted brothers were brought up by the alcoholic parent. This study design would show an effect of environment. The brothers exposed to the alcoholic parent were not at greater risk for alcoholism. In other words, there was no measurable effect of the influence of environment on the development of alcoholism.

Alcoholism is a disease with significant genetic factors underlying its development. Having a parent who is alcoholic does not, however, predetermine your fate. As the author of this study points out, "We can say that even with an alcoholic parent the odds that a man will achieve alcoholic or even problem drinker status are something like three to one against, with at least an even chance that he will be no more than a moderate drinker."[19]

ALCOHOL AND HYPERTENSION

There is an interesting relationship between alcohol consumption and the development of high blood pressure. People who consume two drinks of alcohol per day or less show no association with high blood pressure. In fact, women may actually have a slightly decreased blood pressure.[20]

A large study involving nearly 84,000 people has substantiated other reports that in heavy drinkers, that is, three drinks or more per day, there is a significant relationship between drinking and the development of hypertension.[21] The authors of this study concluded that there is a "strong possibility that regular use of alcohol in amounts above an unknown threshold results in higher blood pressure in a large proportion of persons."

ALCOHOL AND CANCER OF THE HEAD AND NECK

Alcohol consumption is now thought to be an important factor in the development of cancer of the mouth, throat, tongue, and voice box. More than 50 percent of these tumors are causally related to alcohol.[22]

We have stated previously that people who abuse alcohol also tend to be smokers. The combination of alcohol and cigarette smoking magnifies the cancer-inducing effect of either one alone. Thus, alcohol and tobacco, acting jointly, account for 75 percent of these cancers.[23]

It seems likely that the elimination of either risk factor, that is, smoking or drinking, would have a significant impact on the incidence of cancer of the head and neck.

ALCOHOL AND PREGNANCY

Recently, it has been recognizd that the excessive consumption of alcohol during pregnancy can have devastating and lifelong effects on the unborn fetus. In 1973, the so-called Fetal Alcohol Syndrome was described. This was the first acknowledgment of what is now considered to be a significant problem.

Children born to alcoholic mothers have a constellation of defects, including small size, low birth weight, small head size, and significant mental retardation. One-third to one-half of the children of alcoholic mothers will show evidence of these defects; 17 percent are reported to die within the first week of life.[24,25]

Alcohol easily and rapidly crosses the placental and blood-brain barriers of the fetus to achieve blood levels equal to that of the mother.[26] Animal experiments in five species—chicken, rat, mouse, ewe, and guinea pig—have shown similar malformations upon exposure to alcohol. There are reports that occasionally at birth alcohol can be detected on the baby's breath in alcoholic mothers.

There is no evidence concerning how much alcohol is necessary to cause damage to the fetus. Therefore, pregnant women should be aware that there may be danger in drinking only moderate amounts of alcohol.

One of the investigators who originally described the syndrome, David W. Smith, commenting on its serious consequences, stated, "The baby's capabilities are limited, they are limited for life."[27]

PREVENTION

The prevention of alcohol abuse is a difficult but important goal in the United States. In addition to an attack on the problem of current alcoholics, a closer look at preventive intervention in early school years is important. It is in these years, before drinking patterns are established, that intervention may be most successful.

There are many programs of both inpatient and outpatient design that are available to attempt to rehabilitate alcoholics. One of the best known and most widely utilized is Alcoholics Anonymous (AA).

AA was founded in 1935 by two alcoholics, Bill W. and Dr. Bob, in order to provide support and comradeship to fellow problem drinkers who wanted to abstain. Since that beginning, AA has become a world-wide organization with 16,000 groups in the United States and Canada and 12,000 others in some 96 countries around the world.

AA is estimated to reach some 4 percent of the alcoholics in the United States. Members are encouraged to attend at least one meeting per week. At these meetings, individuals relate personal accounts about the difficulties in their lives caused by alcohol. The intimacy of these narratives leads to the formation of strong personal bonds and support structures.

AA is guided by the philosophy contained in the so-called "twelve steps." These steps are:

1. We admitted we were powerless over alcohol—that our lives had become unmanageable.
2. We came to believe that a Power greater than ourselves could restore us to sanity.
3. We made a decision to turn our will and our lives over to the care of God as we understood Him.
4. We made a searching and fearless moral inventory of ourselves.
5. We admitted to God, to ourselves, and to another human being the exact nature of our wrongs.
6. We were entirely ready to have God remove all these defects of character.
7. We humbly asked Him to remove our shortcomings.
8. We made a list of all persons we had harmed and became willing to make amends to them all.

9. We directed amends to such people wherever possible, except when to do so would injure them or others.
10. We continued to take personal inventory and when we were wrong promptly admitted it.
11. We sought through prayer and meditation to improve our conscious contact with God, as we understood him, prayed only for knowledge of His Will for us and the power to carry that out.
12. Having had a spiritual awakening as the result of these steps, we tried to carry this message to alcoholics and practice these principles in all our affairs.

AA groups are located all over the country. Their phone number is listed in the phone book, and they are known for their efforts to help alcoholics looked for aid.

Much work has been done to identify and monitor the drinking problem where it arises: in high schools throughout the country. *The Monitoring the Future Project* is an ongoing nationwide study of high school seniors conducted by the University of Michigan's Institute for Social Research for the National Institute on Drug Abuse. They found, in a recently reported paper, some very interesting correlations between personal and sociologic variables and drug use:[28]

Sex Differences: Females now exceed males in the use of cigarettes; however, males drink more alcohol and use more marijuana.

Racial Comparisons: For all categories of drugs but especially for alcohol, blacks reported less usage than whites. In 1979, more than one-half the black seniors reported no use of alcohol during the previous 30 days, in contrast to about one-fourth of the whites.

Parents' Educational Level: Little correlation with drug use.

Regional Differences: Northeast—above average drug use
South—below average in all drugs except cigarettes
West—below average in cigarettes and alcohol
North Central—average

College Plans: The number of occasions involving heavy alcohol consumption is much lower among the college bound.

Grades: Negative correlation. The worse the grades, the more drug use.

Truancy: Strongly linked to drug usage

Religious Commitment: Negative association with drugs

Political Views: Conservatives used less drugs.

Social Lifestyle: Frequency of dating and going out is correlated with both alcohol and marijuana use.

A recent intervention trial in two California junior high schools was undertaken;[29] 526 students were trained to resist social pressures toward tobacco, alcohol, and drug use. After a 2-year follow-up, there was significantly less smoking, alcohol, and marijuana use in this group.

It is apparent that alcohol abuse is a major problem in the United States. There is some evidence that early preventive intervention trials in junior and senior high schools may be fruitful in preventing the development of deleterious drinking patterns.

Educational efforts on the dangers of alcohol should be encouraged with special attention to high-risk groups like pregnant women. There is no easy solution to a problem as extensive and widespread as this. Awareness is the first step.

REFERENCES

1. Alcoholism—Medical Consequences and Therapy. *U.S. Pharmacist,* June/July 1980, 47–59.
2. Archibald H: Changing drinking patterns in Ontario — Some implications. *Addictions* 20: 2–17, 1973.
3. Alcoholism—Medical Consequences and Therapy. *U.S. Pharmacist,* June/July 1980, 47–59.
4. Poley W, et al: *Alcholism: A Treatment Manual.* New York, Gardner Press, Inc., 1979.
5. Poley W, et al: *Alcholism: A Treatment Manual.* New York, Gardner Press, Inc., 1979.
6. Alcoholism—Medical Consequences and Therapy. *U.S. Pharmacist,* June/July 1980, 47–59.
7. LeDain Gerald: *Final Report of the Commission of Inquiry Into the Non-Medical Use of Drugs.* Ottowa, Queens Printer for Canada, 1973.
8. Brody J, et al: On considering alcohol as a risk factor in specific diseases. *American Journal of Epidemiology* 107:462–466, 1978.
9. Poley W, et al: *Alcholism: A Treatment Manual.* New York, Gardner Press, Inc., 1979.

10. Alcoholism—Medical Consequences and Therapy. *U.S. Pharmacist,* June/July 1980, 47–59.

11. Poley W, et al: *Alcholism: A Treatment Manual.* New York, Gardner Press, Inc., 1979.

12. Brody J, et al: On considering alcohol as a risk factor in specific diseases. *American Journal of Epidemiology* 107: 1978.

13. Poley W, et al: *Alcholism: A Treatment Manual.* New York, Gardner Press, Inc., 1979.

14. Brody J, et al: On considering alcohol as a risk factor in specific diseases. *American Journal of Epidemiology* 107:462–466, 1978.

15. Alcoholism—Medical Consequences and Therapy. *U.S. Pharmacist,* June/July 1980, 47–59.

16. Alcoholism—Medical Consequences and Therapy. *U.S. Pharmacist,* June/July 1980, 47–59.

17. Goodwin D: Hereditary factors in alcoholism. *Hospital Practice,* May 1978, 121–130.

18. Goodwin D: Hereditary factors in alcoholism. *Hospital Practice,* May 1978, 121–130.

19. Goodwin D: Hereditary factors in alcoholism. *Hospital Practice,* May 1978, 121–130.

20. Klatsky A, et al: Alcohol consumption and blood pressure. *New England Journal of Medicine,* May 26, 1977; 1194–1199.

21. Klatsky A, et al: Alcohol consumption and blood pressure. *New England Journal of Medicine,* May 26, 1977; 1194–1199.

22. Rothman K: The effect of alcohol consumption on risk of cancer of the head and neck. *Epidemiology, Carcinogenesis and Virology* 51–55.

23. Rothman K: The effect of alcohol consumption on risk of cancer of the head and neck. *Epidemiology, Carcinogenesis and Virology* 51–55.

24. Poley W, et al: *Alcholism: A Treatment Manual.* New York, Gardner Press, Inc., 1979.

25. Erb L, et al: The fetal alcohol syndrome (FAS). *Clinical Pediatrics* 17:644–649, 1978.

26. Erb L, et al: The fetal alcohol syndrome (FAS). *Clinical Pediatrics* 17:644–649, 1978.

27. Jones KL, et al: Pattern of malformation in offspring of chronic alcoholic mothers. *Lancet* 1: 1267–71, 1973.

28. Bachman J, et al: Smoking, drinking, and drug use among American high school students: correlates and trends 1975–79. *American Journal of Public Health* 71:59–69, 1981.

29. McAlister A, et al: Pilot study of smoking, alcohol and drug abuse prevention. *American Journal of Public Health* 70:59–69, 1980.

FOURTEEN

Coffee

Over the centuries, coffee and tea have been variously praised and condemned as healthful or potentially dangerous beverages. This debate continues even today. Details concerning the origins of the regular ingestion of these beverages has been lost to history. However, one interesting story concerning the discovery of coffee has recently surfaced.[1]

According to legend, it was an Arabian priest who first discovered coffee. Local shepherds noticed that some goats in their flocks would eat the berries of the coffee plant and would stay awake during the night instead of sleeping. The priest, upon learning of this, had the berries made into a beverage that allowed him to stay awake during the night in long hours of devotional prayer.

Whatever its origins, coffee has grown into an immensely popular beverage in the United States. Many believe that the widespread enjoyment of coffee is because of its stimulant or "pick-me-up" effect. If this is indeed the case, it is not without precedent in the rest of the world.

Man has found the tea leaf in China, the kola nut in West Africa, the cocoa bean in Mexico, the ilex plant from which maté is made in Brazil, and the cassina or Christmas berry tree in North America.[2] All of these plants contain caffeine and have been brewed into popular beverages.

At the turn of the century, many believed coffee was an intoxicating drink with potentially serious health hazards that needed to be studied.[3,4] Concern about drug addiction, in particular with the opiates, was rising, and the pharmacologic activity of caffeine was looked on with suspicion. In 1902, Crothers classed morphine use with caffeine use and wrote that caffeine caused a loss of self-control, spells of agitation, and depression and psychotic behavior.[5]

In 1912, public concern over caffeine led the Coca-Cola company to sponsor a study of the effects of caffeine on mental and physical capabilities.[6] A careful and well-controlled study was done that showed that at doses of caffeine from 65 to 139 mg, mostly beneficial mental and physical effects accrued. Higher doses of 390 mg of caffeine were characterized by tremors, insomnia, and poor physical performance.[7]

Despite these early concerns, coffee rapidly became the widely used and culturally accepted beverage that it is today. In order to gain some perspective into coffee's effects on our bodies, a review of its major biologically active component, caffeine, follows.

CAFFEINE

The stimulant action of caffeine is well known. It is this biologic property that has made caffeine a useful component of many over-the-counter and prescription drugs. However, caffeine is a potent drug and actually has many diverse actions upon the body (Table 14-1).

TABLE 14-1. BIOLOGIC EFFECTS OF CAFFEINE

Diuretic (stimulates urination)

Heart muscle stimulant

Brain (stimulates the central nervous system)

Smooth muscle relaxant

Stimulates stomach acid secretion (gastric acid)

Elevates blood sugar and blood fat levels
(plasma glucose and free fatty acids)

TABLE 14-2. DIETARY SOURCES OF CAFFEINE
AND RELATED COMPOUNDS

Food Source		Amount
Coffee	1 cup	85 mg caffeine
Tea	1 cup	50 mg caffeine
		2 mg theobromine
		1 mg theophylline
Cocoa	1 cup	5 mg caffeine
		250 mg theobromine
Cola drinks	10 oz	40 mg caffeine

Adapted from Graham.[8]

In 1972, it is estimated that approximately 34 million lbs of caffeine were consumed by Americans.[8] This large quantity of caffeine was ingested as a natural constituent of coffee, tea, cocoa, and cola soft drinks, as an additive in cola drinks, and in medications (Tables 14-2 and 14-3). Coffee consumption accounted for 75 percent or 25 million lbs of the total caffeine consumed. Tea, responsible for 3.8 million lbs of caffeine intake, ranked a distant second. Cola beverages contributed the least, with approximately one-half their caffeine content coming from the kola nut and an equal amount added by the manufacturers.

Coffee is easily the most important source of caffeine in our diet. Tea and cola supply much lesser amounts of caffeine but together add large quantities of the related compounds theophylline and theobromine. Smaller amounts of caffeine are present in certain foods such as

TABLE 14-3. CAFFEINE CONTENT IN
PRESCRIPTION MEDICATIONS

	Caffeine Present
APC (aspirin, phenacetin, and caffeine)	32 mg
Cafergot	100 mg
Darvon compound	32 mg
Fiorinal	40 mg

coffee-flavored ice cream, chocolate bars, and chocolate-flavored foods.

Caffeine is a plant alkaloid that is structurally very similar to theophylline, a component of tea, and theobromine, a constituent of cocoa. These compounds are thought to possess much of their biologic activity because of their chemical similarity to the important naturally occurring substances known as purines.

Imbibed caffeine is readily absorbed into all parts of the body, metabolized, and excreted into the urine. It is rapidly cleared from the body and has a plasma half life of approximately 3 hours. (Plasma half life is a measure of the rapidity of clearance of a substance from the blood.)

The amount of caffeine present in coffee beans has a wide range of natural variability. Freshly ground roasted coffee can range from 0.8 to 1.8 percent caffeine.[9] The particular variety of plant, its geographic location, altitude, climate, and local cultural practices, all influence the caffeine content of the coffee bean.

The International Coffee Association projected that in 1974, 2.25 cups of coffee were consumed daily by persons 16 years of age or older in the United States. This equates to a daily caffeine intake for most Americans of almost 200 mg from coffee alone. The dose of caffeine usually considered pharmacologically active is 200 mg. Therefore, most Americans consume at or close to pharmacologic doses of caffeine on a daily basis.

COFFEE AND HEART DISEASE

There has been a great deal of public and medical concern about the relationship between coffee drinking and heart attacks. Since the effects of caffeine on the circulation, such as an increase in heart rate, can be readily detected, there has been suspicion over many years of a link between heart attacks and coffee consumption.[10] In recent years, several well-designed studies have explored this hypothesized relationship.

The Boston Collaborative Drug Surveillance Program[11] compared 276 patients who were discharged from the hospital after sustaining a heart attack compared with 1104 control patients. They found that the heart patients gave a history of drinking appreciably more coffee prior to admission than the controls.

A second hospital-based study gave further support to a proposed link between heart attacks and coffee consumption.[12] In this study, 440 patients with diagnosed recent heart attacks were compared to 12,319 patients with other diseases. The authors reported that a history of drinking one to five cups of coffee daily was associated with a 60 percent increase in the risk of heart attacks, whereas the consumption of six or more cups gave rise to an increased risk of approximately 120 percent. Although tea also contains caffeine, they found no association between tea consumption and an increased risk of heart attacks.

Several subsequent studies have failed to confirm these reports. A comparison of 454 heart attack victims and two control groups revealed no correlation between drinking more than six cups of coffee daily and the incidence of first heart attacks.[13] In this study, patients had previously undergone multiphasic health checkups and completed health questionnaires that included questions about coffee consumption. Therefore, information about coffee intake was obtained without the potential bias of an acute stressful situation.

In a subsequent study, the wives of 649 men who had expired as a result of heart disease were questioned about the coffee-consumption habits of their husbands.[14] This was compared to information supplied from the wives of 649 neighborhood controls. These authors concluded that there is little or no risk of death from heart disease associated with coffee consumption.

The large prospective Framingham Study followed 4492 people for a 12-year period and indicated no significant association between coffee drinking and heart disease, heart attack, stroke, chest pain (angina pectoris), or sudden death.[15]

A recently published study examined the relationship of coffee drinking to heart attacks in young women. The researchers reviewed the coffee-drinking habits of 48 patients and 980 controls. They reported no significant association between coffee drinking and heart attacks.[16]

Studies thus far have not established coffee consumption as a risk factor in either heart disease or heart attacks.

COFFEE AND PALPITATIONS

It has been widely believed, mostly on anecdotal evidence, that coffee and other caffeine-containing beverages can trigger palpitations and extra heart beat.[17] From a pharmacologic point of view, it is known that large doses of caffeine can directly stimulate the heart muscle to produce rapid heart rates.[18] In a recent study, a stomach tube was passed into volunteers. These individuals received either caffeine or placebo solutions variously. It was found that caffeine could produce symptoms that included rapid heart rates and palpitations.[19]

A large population study screened 7311 men aged 37 to 57 who had no history of heart disease to determine the relationship of palpitations to food, drink, cigarette smoking, and sleep habits.[20] This recent study found that heavy coffee consumption, that is, more than nine cups per day, was associated with more than twice the likelihood of extra heart beats being present at any age compared to light (two cups or less) or no coffee consumption.

It is apparent that there is a relationship between heavy coffee consumption and palpitations. There is no evidence that this is a dangerous phenomenon when not in the setting of a recent heart attack. Previously mentioned studies show no relationship between coffee consumption and either sudden death or death from heart disease (both of which might be thought attributable to abnormal electrical heart rhythms). Although palpitations do occur more readily in people who drink large amounts of coffee, their clinical significance, if any, is not established.

COFFEE AND STOMACH PROBLEMS

Coffee has been associated with a variety of stomach and gastrointestinal problems, including peptic or duodenal ulcers, hiatal hernia, and diarrhea. In fact, these associations have never been proved. Many of these effects were thought to occur because of the known pharmacologic activity of caffeine. In this case, as has been aptly stated, coffee is more than tasty caffeine.

Coffee was thought to be associated with peptic ulcer disease because of its ability to increase gastric acid secretion. However, a variety of studies have failed to establish a cause and effect relationship between coffee consumption and either the induction or exacerbation of peptic ulcer disease.[25] In an interesting and unexpected finding, one study found that both regular and decaffeinated coffee have virtually the same effects on stomach acid secretion.[22]

A recently published study examined the effects of coffee intake on several variables (stomach acid secretion and muscle tone in the lower end of the feeding tube) in 31 people who had modified coffee intake because of gastrointestinal symptoms.[23] Heartburn was not due to any intrinsic harmful components in coffee but related to underlying abnormalities in these people.

There is no evidence that supports the concept that coffee is a risk factor in peptic ulcer disease, hiatal hernia, diabetes, or any other gastrointestinal problem. Furthermore, there is no apparent difference in effect on the stomach with either caffeinated or decaffeinated coffee.

COFFEE AND BLADDER CANCER

Coffee has been found in several studies in the past to have a weak association with the development of bladder cancer. These studies were unable to demonstrate any dose-response relationship between the amount of coffee consumed and the incidence of this disease.[24-26]

Recently, other studies have examined this relationship. In one study of 569 bladder cancer patients, data on dietary habits, employment, and tobacco use were obtained.[27] Some elevation of risk was found in those who consumed large amounts of coffee. A Canadian study of 480 males and 152 females with bladder cancer has been reported.[28] The authors noted a slight increase in bladder cancer risk for males consuming all types of coffee, including regular and instant, and for females consuming instant coffee. They could not establish a dose-response relationship.

There is apparently a weak association between the use of coffee and the development of bladder cancer.

COFFEE AND CANCER OF THE PANCREAS

The possibility of a link between cancer of the pancreas and coffee consumption has drawn much recent attention. This possibility is of particular significance when we consider that cancer of the pancreas is the fourth most common fatal cancer in the United States.

A recent case report from Australia stirred a good deal of interest in the medical community.[29] The authors report the virtual simultaneous occurrence of cancer of the pancreas in a husband and wife.

Both of these individuals shared two peculiar dietary idiosyncrasies:

1. They ingested large amounts of margarine, in which they cooked all their food. After the food was cooked, they would pour the remaining margarine, now a thick sauce, over the food.
2. They routinely added "coffee syrup," a liquid concentrate of coffee, to their ground coffee before percolation. This is a not uncommon practice in some parts of Europe.

The authors of this report suggested that the utilization of this coffee syrup may have played a possible causative role in the development of cancer of the pancreas.

A recently published study from the Department of Epidemiology at Harvard has caused a great deal of public and medical reaction.[30] The authors report that coffee consumption is associated with an increased risk of pancreatic cancer. The results of their study indicated that an individual who drinks one to two cups of coffee daily has increased his risk of developing pancreas cancer 1.8 times. Those who drink three to four cups daily increase their risk 2.7 times. They conclude that the portion of pancreas cancer associated with coffee consumption may be greater than 50 percent.

However, this study has not met universal acceptance. Careful analysis reveals that there are several potential design flaws that may invalidate these results. Some of the problems with the study include:

1. The study was not originally designed to study the influence of coffee on pancreas cancer. It was designed to reevaluate relationships between cancer of the pancreas with tobacco and alcohol. Data on coffee and tea consumption were obtained in an incidental way.
2. In the selection of the control group, diseases associated with tobacco and alcohol were excluded. However, there is a known relationship between both coffee consumption and alcohol and tobacco use. Therefore, the selection of the control group actually eliminated from analysis people who were more likely to drink coffee.
3. Many patients in the control group had gastrointestinal diseases such as gastritis, colitis, etc. These patients might very

well have been told to lessen their coffee consumption, or they may have done so of their own volition.

4. Cases for the study were gathered from 11 different hospitals over a 5-year period. The pathologic diagnosis of cancer of the pancreas has been repeatedly shown to be difficult and a potential source of error in such studies.[31] This error can only be exacerbated in cases taken from this large a number of institutions.

5. The retrospective design technique is in general a less well regarded study design than a prospective study.

The National Cancer Institute, commenting on this study's findings, stated, "Caution should be exercised regarding overreacting to a preliminary finding until results of further studies are reported...."[32]

The question of a relationship between coffee consumption and cancer of the pancreas has been raised. It appears that further studies are required to either confirm or deny any such relationship.

COFFEE AND PSYCHOLOGICAL EFFECTS

Caffeine is known to have major psychotropic effects (effects on behavior). Its stimulant actions were utilized in early attempts to treat depression with drugs. However, it soon became apparent that there frequently was a rebound depression associated with its use.

Coffee consumption, either in particularly susceptible individuals or in large users of the beverage, has been reported to trigger symptoms virtually indistinguishable from severe anxiety neuroses.[33] Caffeine intoxication, corresponding to ten cups of coffee over several hours, has been described as producing tremulousness and frank delirium.[34]

These effects of large amounts of coffee intake have inspired a very interesting study.[35] Psychiatric inpatients in many North American hospitals consume large quantities of coffee and tea. This is thought to occur partly because of boredom and partly to counteract the sedative effects of the medication they are taking. In a study of psychiatric inpatients, the effect of the elimination of caffeine intake was studied. Coffee on the wards was changed to the decaffeinated variety without the knowledge of either patients or staff. It was found that there was a general improvement in those patients who exhibited less anxiety, irritability, and hostility. Upon a resumption of regular (ie, caffeinated) coffee use, the improvement was promptly reversed.

Caffeine-withdrawal headaches are an important but frequently ignored type of headache.[36] It is commonly a severe headache, and individuals with this syndrome are often anxious or depressed. They feel "less healthy" and have a significantly higher caffeine intake than persons without such headaches.

We have discussed a wide range of diseases and their association with coffee intake (Table 14-4 through 14-6). Perhaps the major effect of coffee consumption on Americans is to be found in its psychological consequences. Many Americans have switched to decaffeinated coffee for these reasons. At this point, it seems reasonable to say that moderate consumption of coffee, either caffeinated or decaffeinated, does not seem to pose any particular hazard to most people.

TABLE 14-4. COFFEE AS A RISK FACTOR

Palpitations (cardiac arrhythmias)

Bladder cancer

Anxiety neurosis

Depression

TABLE 14-5. COFFEE AS A POSSIBLE RISK FACTOR

Cancer of the pancreas

TABLE 14-6. COFFEE IS NOT A RISK FACTOR

Peptic ulcers (duodenal ulcers)

Hiatal hernia

Diarrhea

Heart disease and heart attacks

Sudden death from heart attacks

REFERENCES

1. Ritchie J: Central nervous system stimulants, II. *The Zanthines, chap 19. The Pharmacological Basis of Therapeutics,* ed. 3 New York, Goodman and Gilman, 1965, p. 354.

2. Stephenson P: Physiologic and psychotropic effects of caffeine on man, *Journal of the American Dietetic Assocation* 71:240–247, 1977.

3. Stephenson P: Physiologic and psychotropic effects of caffeine on man, *Journal of the American Dietetic Assocation* 71:240–247, 1977.

4. Graham D: Caffeine — its identity, dietary sources, intake and biological effects. *Nutrition Reviews* 36: 97–102, 1978.

5. Crothers T: *Morphinism and Narcomanias from Other Drugs.* Philadelphia, Saunders, 1902.

6. Stephenson P: Physiologic and psychotropic effects of caffeine on man, *Journal of the American Dietetic Assocation* 71:240–247, 1977.

7. Hollingsworth H: The influence of caffeine on mental and motor efficiency. *Archives of Psychology* 22: 1, 1912.

8. Graham D: Caffeine — its identity, dietary sources, intake and biological effects. *Nutrition Reviews* 36: 97–102, 1978.

9. Graham D: Caffeine — its identity, dietary sources, intake and biologica' effects. *Nutrition Reviews* 36: 97–102, 1978.

10. Coffee and Cardiovascular Disease. *The Medical Letter,* August 12, 1977.

11. *Lancet* 2:1279, 1972.

12. Jick H, et al: *New England Journal of Medicine* 289:63, 1973.

13. Klatsky A, et al: *JAMA* 226:540, 1973.

14. Hennekens C, et al: *New England Journal of Medicine* 294:633, 1976.

15. Dawber T, et al: *New England Journal of Medicine* 291:871, 1974.

16. Rosenberg L, et al: Coffee drinking, and myocardial infarction in young women. *American Journal of Epidemiology* 111:1980.

17. Caffeinated drinks: public health problem. Newland S (ed): *Connecticut Medicine* 43:331–332, 1979.

18. Rosenberg L: Coffee drinking and myocardial infarction in young men. *Amerian Journal of Epidemiology,* 111:675–681, 1980.

19. Finn R, et al: *Lancet* 1978, 1:426.

20. Prineast R, et al: Coffee, tea and VPB. *Journal of Chronic Diseases.* 33: 67–72, 1979.

21. Select Committee on GRAS Substances: *Tentative Evaluation of the Health Aspects of Caffeine as a Food Ingredient (SCEGS-89).* Bethesda, Maryland, Life Sciences Research Office, Federation of American Societies for Experimental Biology, 1976.

22. Cohen S, et al: Gastric acid secretion and lower-esophageal sphincter pressure in response to coffee and caffeine. *New England Journal of Medicine* 293: 897, 1975.
23. Cohen S: Journal of pathogenesis of coffee-induced gastrointestinal symptoms. *New England Journal of Medicine* 303:122–124, 1980.
24. Dunham L, et al: Rates, interview, and pathology study of cancer of urinary bladder in New Orleans, LA. *Journal of National Cancer Institute* 41:683–709, 1968.
25. Cole P: Coffee drinking and cancer of the lower urinary tract. *Lancet* 1:1335–1337, 1971.
26. Simon D: Coffee drinking and cancer of the lower urinary tract. *Journal of the National Cancer Institute* 54:587–591, 1975.
27. Mettlin C, et al: Dietary risk factors in human bladder cancer. *American Journal of Epidemilogy* 110:255–263, 1979.
28. Howe G, et al: Tobacco use, occupation, coffee, various nutrients, and bladder cancer, *Journal of the National Cancer Institute*, 64:1980.
29. Ferguson L, et al: Simultaneous cancer of the pancreas occurring in husband and wife. *Gut* 2:537–540, 1980.
30. MacMahon B, et al: Coffee and cancer of the pancreas, *New England Journal of Medicine* 630–633, 1981.
31. Mach T: Epidemiology of pancreas cancer in Los Angeles, *Cancer* 47:1474–1483, 1981.
32. Coffee and Cancer: A Brewing Concern. *Science News*, March 21, 1981, p. 181.
33. Greden J: Anxiety or caffeinism? A diagnostic dilemma. *American Journal of Psychiatry*, 131:1089–1092, 1974.
34. Pierce C, et al: *American Journal of Psychiatry*, 438, 1978.
35. De Freitas B, et al: Effects of caffeine in chronic psychiatric patients. *American Journal of Psychiatry* 136:10, 1979.
36. Greden J, et al: Caffeine-withdrawal headache: a clinical profile. *Psychosomatics* 21: 1980.